3 Bi-Sexual Comedies

Plus an Assortment of Plays

Norman Beim

AF271175

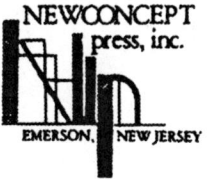

NEWCONCEPT
press, inc.

EMERSON, NEW JERSEY

NEW CONCEPT PRESS
425 West 57th Street   Suite 2J
New York, New York 10019
212-265-6284
Fax: 212-265-6659
newconpres@aol.com

All inquiries for performance rights should be addressed to:
Samuel French, Inc
45 West 25th Street
New York,New York 10010
212-206-8990

Library of Congress Control Number:2013912372

Beim Norman
3 bi-sexual comedies plus an assortment of plays:
come out, come out wherever you are: love among the artists:
the road not taken: choices: the proper technique: politics as
usual, kidding around, fancy meeting you

ISBN: (ALK, paper) 978-0931231-22-3, 0-931231-22-1

1.Drama 1.Title: 3 Bi-Sexual Comedies, Plus An Assortment of
Plays

Special thanks to: Larry Erlbaum, Frank Bara, Marty Beim,

Printed in The United States
10 9 8 7 6 5 4 3 2 1

TABLE OF CONTENTS

Come Out, Come Out, Wherever You Are   Page 1

Love Among The Artists   Page 51

The Road Not Taken   Page 105

Choices   Page 159

The Proper Technique   Page 221

Politics As Usual   Page 305

Kidding Around   Page 327

Fancy Meeting You   Page 345

QUERY

Relationship between the sexes has always puzzled me. The mystery began when, at the age of eleven or twelve, male relatives, when they visited, stopped kissing me. They continued to kiss my sister, but not me. At first I was offended. Then I wondered if I'd done anything wrong. Then I observed that men never kissed one another. They just shook hands. I gathered that that must be the custom.

As an adolescent my romantic dreams involved falling in love with a beautiful girl, getting married and living in a penthouse overlooking the New York skyline. I also admired beauty in a male, and I wondered if that was wrong.

I was thirteen when a friend gathered a group of us in the cellar of my house and introduced us to the art of masturbation. I had a difficult time arriving at whatever I was supposed to arrive at. One of my friends reached out and offered to assist me, but I refused his help. I can do it myself, I thought. I'm not that dumb.

And then I read about homosexuality and heterosexuality; and I noticed two classmates who seemed terribly close, and I concluded that they must be homosexuals. One boy in our group gathered some of us and led us to the house of one of the boys, and some of us called out his name in a taunting manner. I didn't think that was very nice, and I just stood there, feeling terribly guilty. The boy's sister came out of the house, looked directly at me and said, "Norman, you're a nice boy. Why don't you leave my brother alone?" I slunk away, ashamed, followed by the other boys.

And I wondered. There are very macho men in prison, carrying on with other men. And, suppose a male, who was supposed to be homosexual, was alone with a woman on a desert island, wouldn't he finally end up having sex with the woman, and wouldn't that end up being a pleasant experience? And might that not be a habit, after being rescued, that he might want to continue...or not? Could it be that we are all bi-sexual...on a sliding scale perhaps?

But the purpose of sex is to reproduce, isn't it? Why this constant urge? It's all very confusing.

COME OUT, COME OUT, WHEREVER YOU ARE
A Bi-Sexual Comedy In Two Acts

CAST OF CHARACTERS

Lily Byington

Joshua Byington

Edith Byington

Hal Billingsley

Drew Timmons

Marian Short

SCENE
Living room of the Byington home,
in a small university town in New England

ACT ONE

Scene One

(The living room. An early summer evening. LILY, a well-preserved woman in her fifties, wearing an evening gown, enters angrily from the dining room. JOSHUA, a scholarly looking man in his fifties, in a tuxedo, enters from upstairs holding his tie.)

JOSHUA: What's the matter now?

LILY: It's Marian. She refuses to wear the shoes I bought her.

JOSHUA: She's wearing the uniform, isn't she?

LILY: You think I'm ridiculous, I know, just because I have certain principles.

JOSHUA: Principles is it?

LILY: Yes, principles. Why shouldn't we dress for dinner? Why shouldn't we look as attractive as we possibly can? I shall never forget, as long as I live, when we went to the theatre last month in New York, that man, in his undershirt...

JOSHUA: Was it an undershirt?

LILY: It most certainly was an undershirt, and a soiled one at that.

(JOSHUA holds out his tie.)

LILY: Oh, all right. *(LILY accepts the tie and proceeds to tie it for him.)* What are you smiling at? You know perfectly well how to tie this tie.

JOSHUA: Not as well as you do, my dear. Is Brenda coming too?

1

COME OUT, COME OUT, WHEREVER YOU ARE

LILY: No. She had a previous engagement.

JOSHUA: Why can't you accept her?

LILY: Once and for all, I have nothing against Brenda. Our daughter is perfectly free to love whomever she chooses. The fact of the matter is, Edith is still in love with Kenneth, the memory of that dear dead boy, at any rate.

JOSHUA: I see. So you're firmly convinced that Edith is basically heterosexual,

LILY: Basically this, basically that. Kenneth's death left Edith broken hearted, and Brenda just happened to provide the love she needed at a time when she was open and vulnerable.

JOSHUA: You really should be teaching psychology.

LILY: As a matter of fact, I'd probably be a very valuable addition to your psychology department.

JOSHUA: Now don't you go running down our faculty.

LILY: Yes, well, there's one member of your faculty who could use some guidance.

JOSHUA: You're referring to Drew, of course.

LILY: If Kenneth hadn't come along, I really think that she and Drew would might have hit it off.

JOSHUA: Quite possibly.

LILY: And Drew is still an eligible bachelor.

JOSHUA; So he is.

COME OUT, COME OUT, WHEREVER YOU ARE

LILY: And I do think he's finally at the point where's he's ready to settle down.

JOSHUA: So you've invited him to take Brenda's place.

.LILY: Unfortunately Drew wasn't sure he could make it, so I've invited Hal Billingsley as well.

JOSHUA: Hal Billingsley?

LILY: Yes, Hal Billingsley. What's wrong with Hal Billingsley?

JOSHUA: Hal Billingsley is a rather simple soul, and I sincerely doubt if Hal owns a tuxedo.

LILY: Just listen to yourself. And you accuse me of being a snob.

JOSHUA: Well I, for one, am not going to embarrass that poor man. I'm getting out of this monkey suit. That's what we peasants sometimes call it.

> *(LILY starts off.)*

JOSHUA: Where are you going?

LILY: I'm going to call Hal Billingsley.

> *(JOSHUA heaves a sigh and shakes his head as LILY goes off.)*

LILY: *(Offstage, after a moment)* Hello? Hello, Billy, dear. Can I speak to your father? I see. No, no. Never mind. *(SHE reenters.)* Hal's on his way. Well, if you're going to change, then I'll have to change as well. And what about Edith?

COME OUT, COME OUT, WHEREVER YOU ARE

(EDITH, an attractive woman in her mid-thirties, wearing an evening gown, enters.)

EDITH: What about Edith?

LILY: Good lord, Edith, you gave me a start! Why didn't you ring the bell?

EDITH: I'm not in the habit of ringing the doorbell of a house I grew up in. What's happening?

LILY: Drew wasn't sure he could make it, so I've invited Hal Billingsley as well.

EDITH: Hal Billingsley. I've always been rather fond of Hal.

LILY: So there you are.

JOSHUA: And your mother's convinced that Hal is going to show up in black tie.

EDITH: Did you tell him that we dress for dinner? Mother dear, in those vintage films you're addicted to, Myrna Loy and William Powell dressed for dinner.

LILY: And so did Clark Gable, and he was quite down to earth.

EDTITH: And you see Hal Billingsley as Clark Gable?

LILY: No, as a matter of fact, I think he's more like Gary Cooper.

JOSHUA: Well, I don't think we ought to embarrass the man by appearing in formal clothes.

EDITH: I quite agree. I'm going back and change.

COME OUT, COME OUT, WHEREVER YOU ARE

LILY: Oh, very well. If you both insist. And there's no need for you to go back. You still have some clothes upstairs. I'll dig them out for you. *(SHE goes off.)*

EDITH: What would she do without those DVDs?

JOSHUA: Actually most of those old movies are better than the ones we have today. They're more succinct, and the violence, as I recall, is not as relentless. What's Brenda up to this evening?

EDITH: I haven't the vaguest idea. The fact of the matter is, Brenda feels that she's not welcome here. Oh, it's not you. It's Mother. *(After a moment SHE smiles.)* Hal Billingsley. He's really a very sweet man. I felt so sorry for him when he lost his wife.

JOSHUA: How long has it been?

EDITH: Three years, It was just about the same time that we received word about Kenny. What happened to Drew, by the way?

JOSHUA: I haven't the vaguest idea. Your mother arranges these things. And now she's upset with Marian.

EDITH: What's wrong with Marian?

JOSHUA: Marian doesn't want to wear the shoes she bought her.

EDITH: She bought her shoes?

JOSHUA: To go with the fancy uniform. She saw this movie with...I think it was Carole Lombard, and the maid wore a fancy uniform, so she thought that Marian should have a fancy uniform. It's interesting how the world evolves. I remember when the word "gay" meant happy, lively. Why don't you have a talk with Marian? Maybe she'll listen to you.

COME OUT, COME OUT, WHEREVER YOU ARE

EDITH: Marian does have a mind of her own.

JOSHUA: She's always been fond of you. It's worth a try.

> *(EDITH heaves a sigh and goes off. LILY enters, wearing an ordinary dress.)*

LILY: Where's she gone to now?

JOSHUA: She's gone to talk to Marian into wearing the shoes. What happened to Drew, by the way? Why did he cancel?

LILY: Did I say he canceled?

> *(EDITH reenters.)*

EDITH: Marian's agreed to wear the shoes this one time.

LILY: Thank you, dear. *(SHE turns to JOSHUA.)* Are you going to change or aren't you?

JOSHUA: I'm going to change. Excuse me. *(HE goes off.)*

LILY: I found a dress for you. That blue one; the one you wore to our anniversary party. I think it'll still fit.

EDITH: Thank you.

LILY: What happened to Brenda?

EDITH: You don't like Brenda, do you?

LILY: I don't dislike Brenda. As a matter of fact, I think she has many admirable qualities. She runs the administration office with an iron hand. And I think her concern for stray animals, cats and dogs, that is, is very touching. And I'm very grateful to her for the love and understanding she's shown you, when you were sorely in need of love and understanding, and if she makes you happy, then I'm happy for you.

EDITH: I see. Are you planning to go abroad this year?

LILY: Your father's going to London. He's working on a book about Pinter, and he's been corresponding with his widow, Lady Antonia Fraser. I'd like to go to Paris.

EDITH: Why don't you

LILY: Alone? Paris is a city for lovers. What are you smiling at? We're not dead, you know. And don't fool yourself, my dear. Your father may be stuffy at times...but not always.

EDITH: I need a drink. Would you like some wine?

LILY: Oh, dear. *(SHE runs off.)*

EDITH: Where are you going?

> *(EDITH shakes her head, sighs, pours a glass of wine and takes a sip. LILY reenters with a small package.)*

LILY: This book your father ordered arrived this morning, and I forgot to tell him. He's getting so forgetful.

> *(JOSHUA reenters wearing a sports jacket.)*

JOSHUA: What's that you've got there?

LILY: The book you ordered.

JOSHUA: *(To EDITH)* Aren't you going to change?

COME OUT, COME OUT, WHEREVER YOU ARE

EDITH: I guess I'd better, since you have.

(EDTITH sets down her glass and goes off.)

JOSHUA: It must be the new book about Pinter. I ordered it weeks ago. *(HE unwraps the package.)* It's a biography of Jean Paul Sartre.

LILY: You can always return it.

JOSHUA: That's not the point. I want to read the Pinter book before I meet with Lady Antonia.

LILY: What you see in Pinter, with all those pauses...

EDITH: *(Offstage)* Mother, would you please come up here? I can't find that dress.

(The doorbell rings.)

LILY: Oh, Lord!

JOSHUA: I'll get it.

(LILY goes off. JOSHUA goes to answer the door.)

JOSHUA: *(Offstage)* Hello, Hal. Come on in.

(HAL BILLINGSLEY, a pleasant looking, solidly built man in his forties, wearing a tuxedo, enters followed by Joshua.)

HAL: Is there anything wrong? You looked at me sort of strange.

JOSHUA: No, no, no.

COME OUT, COME OUT, WHEREVER YOU ARE

HAL: I guess I do look sort of funny in this monkey suit. I only wore it that one time.

JOSHUA: When was that?

HAL: When I got married. Am I too early?

JOSHUA: What's that? No, no. I was just about to go up and change. Can I get you a drink?

HAL: A beer'd be fine...or a coke.

JOSHUA: Actually, I think there may be some beer in the refrigerator.

HAL: You go on ahead and change. Don't you worry about me.

JOSHUA: The beer first.

> *(JOSHUA goes off. HAL takes in the room. After a moment LILY enters. JOSHUA enters with a bottle of beer.)*

JOSHUA: Lily? I thought you were going upstairs to change. That's all right. I'll go first. *(HE hands the beer to Hal.)* Excuse me. *(HE goes off.)*

LILY: How are you, Hal?

HAL: I'm fine, Mrs. Byington. And you?

LILY: A little confused, as you can see. All these last minute changes. It was kind of you to come.

HAL: It was kind of you to invite me. I'm a great admirer of Professor Byington, ever since I heard him speak about English literature.

COME OUT, COME OUT, WHEREVER YOU ARE

LILY: Oh? Are you interested in English literature?

HAL: I like to read about all sorts of things. I guess curious is the word.

LILY: Eclectic.

HAL: If you say so.

LILY: Let me get you a glass for that beer. *(SHE hands him a glass.)*

HAL: Actually I could use an opener.

LILY: Oh, dear *(SHE finds an opener at the bar and hands it to HAL.)* Here you are, dear.

HAL: Thank you. If you wanna go up and change, don't you worry about me.

LILY: It's all this last minute rush.

HAL: I should have just come in an ordinary suit. It would have saved us a lot of trouble. But I know that you and Professor Byington always dress up for dinner.

LILY: How's your little boy by the way?

HAL: He's not that little anymore. He'll be eleven next month.

LILY; My, my, my. It must be difficult for you, bringing up a child all by yourself.

HAL: It ain't easy, Ma'am.

(EDITH enters in her evening gown.)

COME OUT, COME OUT, WHEREVER YOU ARE

EDITH: Good evening, Hal.

HAL: Good evening.

LILY: If you'll excuse me. I'll go up and change. *(SHE goes off.)*

HAL: I guess I came a little too early.

EDITH: It's good of you to join us at the very last minute.

HAL: Glad to oblige. I don't get out that much these days.

EDITH: How's Billy doing?

HAL: He's growing up, that's for sure. Another couple years, he'll be going to high school.

EDITH: Has he shown any special interests?

HAL: Not really, that I know of. But I've been thinking I'd like to try to send him to college. I never bothered, and I sort of regret it.

EDITH: Is there any subject he does well in?

HAL: He's a pretty good student.

EDITH: There are certain aptitude tests he can take, to find out what field he might do well in.

HAL: Oh?

EDITH: I'll look into it for you, and let you know.

HAL: Thank you. I'd appreciate that. As a matter of fact, I've been meaning to get in touch with you.

COME OUT, COME OUT, WHEREVER YOU ARE

EDITH: Oh?

HAL: I came across this snapshot of me and Kenny, just before he went off to war. We were both on the basketball team, you know.

EDITH: Yes, I know.

HAL: I would have joined up with him, but I had a wife and a kid on the way. He was a fine man, Kenny was.

EDITH: Yes, he was.

HAL: I should have brought it with me, that snapshot I mean. I put it aside, 'cause I thought you might like to have it.

EDITH: That's very kind of you. Yes, I would like to have it.

HAL: I'll make a note for myself to drop it off.

EDITH: Thank you. I'd appreciate that.

HAL: It's not easy losing someone you care deeply about.

EDITH: How do you manage?

HAL: You just carry on, I guess. And I do have a responsibility. And you have your teaching, and Miss Lewis, of course. A special friend can sure come in handy.

EDITH: Do you have any special friend?

HAL: No one special, no. But I do have friends. That's the advantage of living in a small town, I guess.

(LILY and JOSHUA reenter in formal attire.)

12

COME OUT, COME OUT, WHEREVER YOU ARE

LILY: Well, I think it's time we sat down to dinner. Edith, why don't you and Hal lead the way. *(To Hal)* You can take your beer if you like.

HAL: Thank you.

(HAL picks up his beer and follows EDITH off.)

JOSHUA: I thought you invited Drew.

LILY: So I did.

JOSHUA: Well, don't you think...?

LILY: No. Just leave things to me dear.

(LILY starts off, follow by JOSHUA as the phone rings.)

JOSHUA: I'll get that.

LILY: No, dear. I'll get it. *(SHE goes off.)* Hello? Drew, dear. We were just about to sit down to dinner. No, no, no. You can join us for coffee. See you later, dear.

(SHE reenters. JOSHUA shakes his head.)

LILY: What?

JOSHUA: Nothing.

(JOSHUA sighs, shakes his head, and offers his arm. LILY takes it, and HE leads her off as the lights come down.)

Scene Two

(Half an hour later. DREW TIMMONS, a polished, attractive man in his middle thirties, is discovered drinking a brandy. He wears a tuxedo. MARIAN SHORT, a solidly built woman of forty or so, enters with a coffee tray which SHE sets down on the sideboard. MARIAN wears a maid's uniform.)

MARIAN: You missed a good dinner.

DREW: Where'd you get that fancy uniform?

MARIAN: That woman gets nuttier by the day.

DREW: Most of us accept life as it is. Mrs. Byington prefers to live life as she thinks it ought to be. So, Marian, how's your love life these days?

MARIAN: Not as interesting as yours, Professor. We haven't seen much of you lately.

DREW: I've been rather busy.

MARIAN: So I gather.

DREW: Oh?

MARIAN: It's a mighty small town. Roger misses you.

DREW: How is your nephew, by the way?

MARIAN: If you must know, he's started to drink again.

DREW: I'm sorry to hear that.

MARIAN: I'm worried about him, Professor. The fact of the matter is, that young man happens to be in love with you.

14

COME OUT, COME OUT, WHEREVER YOU ARE

DREW: Nonsense.

MARIAN: I think it would help if you gave him a call.

DREW: I did what I could for Roger. I got him a job in the mail room, didn't I?

MARIAN: Is that all you did for him?

(LILY enters.)

LILY: Oh, Marian...

MARIAN: Yes, Ma'am?

LILY: There are only four cups.

MARIAN: So there is.

LILY: Would you mind...bringing another cup?

MARIAN: Whatever you say...ma'am. *(SHE goes off.)*

LILY: Well, I'm so glad you could make it.

DREW: Your wish is my command.

LILY: You're such a busy man. That's quite all right, my dear. you're not the only pebble on the beach.

DREW: Oh?

LILY: Hal Billingsley was available.

DREW: Hal Billingsley.

COME OUT, COME OUT, WHEREVER YOU ARE

LILY: Charming man.

DREW: Is this dinner anything special?

LILY: I think Edith needs some cheering up.

DREW: Oh? Are the ladies having any problems?

LILY: Quite possibly.

(*MARIAN reenters with cup and saucer.*)

MARIAN: Are you gonna to eat your dessert, or shall I start to clear?

LILY: Thank you, Marian.

(*MARIAN stands, waiting patiently. LILY snorts and strides off.*)

MARIAN: (*SHE places the cup and saucer on the tray, and turns to DREW.*) Why don't you think about what I said.

DREW: What's that?

MARIAN: My nephew, Roger. Why don't you give him a call.

(*MARIAN hesitates, then goes off. DREW stands, lost in thought, sighs, then goes to the bar, refills his drink, and sits thoughtfully. JOSHUA enters.*)

JOSHUA: Here you are, all by yourself.

DREW: What's that? Yes, well, that's my demerit, for being tardy.

JOSHUA: Oh, that's quite all right. You've been replaced.

16

COME OUT, COME OUT, WHEREVER YOU ARE

DREW: So I gather. But then I thought I was supposed to be the replacement. Is there trouble on the Isle of Lesbos?

JOSHUA: Lily seems to think so. And how's Madame X these days?

DREW: I've come to the alarming conclusion that I've been doing the cuckold a favor.

JOSHUA: Freedom, dear boy, can sometimes be a burden.

(EDITH enters with HAL.)

DREW: Mr. Billingsley.

HAL: Mr. Timmons.

DREW: Thank you for standing in for me.

HAL: Actually, I've been sitting down most of the time.

EDITH: Would you care for some coffee, Drew?

DREW: Not right now, thank you.

EDITH: Daddy?

JOSHUA: Yes, indeed.

EDITH: *(SHE pours coffee.)* Hal?

HAL: Milk and sugar. Two sugars. Thank you.

EDITH: *(SHE hands JOSHUA his coffee and pours coffee for HAL.)* We've been discussing sexuality.

COME OUT, COME OUT, WHEREVER YOU ARE

DREW: Over the appetizer or the entree?

EDITH: Over the chicken soup.

DREW: That's usually the cure for everything, isn't it? And what conclusion have you come to?

JOSHUA: Hal seems to think it all depends on whether the matching paraphernalia fit properly.

(EDITH hands HAL his coffee, then pours one for herself.)

HAL: Thank you.

DREW: It all comes down to mechanics Is that it?

HAL: I was just speaking from my own rather limited experience.

DREW: Sexuality, it seems to me, is a rather complicated area. There's the physical; there's the sentiment, usually referred to as the heart, and then there's the mind.

EDITH: It seems to me that it all has to do with love.

DREW: And the sexual act?

EDITH: Is an expression of love.

DREW: Is it really? As a fallen away Catholic I've been encouraged to believe that the sexual act is a violent assault one is permitted to inflict only upon the person one is promised to.

EDITH: And what conclusion have **you** come to?

DREW: As far as I'm concerned, sexuality is a mystery, just like the existence of God...or electricity...or the universe. It's a subject much too confusing, and much too profound to fathom.

HAL: So why not relax and enjoy it.

DREW: Here, here.

(LILY enters.)

LILY: *(To JOSHUA)* I thought you were going to work on your speech.

JOSHUA: We have guests.

LILY: Guests?! We're family and friends.

DREW: Have you decided what you're going to say to those about to enter the world at large?

JOSHUA: In spite of the economy, in spite of wars and in spite of unemployment?

LILY: I'm sure the professor will be his usual eloquent self if, that is, he prepares his speech properly.

JOSHUA: I'm being banished to my study. If you'll excuse me.

EDITH: Don't work too hard.

(EDITH kisses JOSHUA on the cheek and HE goes off.)

DREW: You're something of a bully, Mrs. Byington.

LILY: Most men require bullying and, if truth were known, they enjoy it. Hal, you promised to build a stand for those plants of mine.

COME OUT, COME OUT, WHEREVER YOU ARE

HAL: I'll need to take some measurements.

LILY: *(To DREW and EDITH)* You'll excuse us, won't you?

EDITH: Do we have any choice?

(HAL follows LILY off.)

EDITH: I envy her, really I do. She's reached a point in life where she's at peace with the world. Oh, I know, I know. She complains about this and she complains about that, but that's part of the joy, this righteous indignation. It keeps her juices flowing.

DREW: How are you and Brenda getting along?

EDITH: I'm fond of Brenda, I really am.

DREW: But you're not in love with her.

EDITH: In love...what does that mean? Romantic passion? And how long does that last? You wake up one morning, and you look at one another, and you ask yourself, Is this the person I want to spend the rest of my life with?

DREW: And what was the answer?

EDITH: That's just the trouble, doctor. I haven't found the answer. And you? You're like the sphinx, mysterious and poker-faced.

DREW: I don't want you to see how frivolous I really am.

EDITH: Why?

DREW: Because I respect you, and I don't want to lose your respect.

COME OUT, COME OUT, WHEREVER YOU ARE

EDITH: You're ashamed of your behavior. Is that it?

DREW: Well, yes, sort of.

EDITH: After the example I've set? A flaming lesbian?

DREW: Are you a flaming lesbian?

EDITH: I have become a poster girl for the local sisterhood. They claim me as their own.

DREW: And are they mistaken?

EDITH: Obviously my current lover is a woman.

DREW: Current? Is she the first in line?

EDITH: The fact is, I fell in love with Brenda, at least I think it was love, and she happened to be a woman.

DREW: It's the person.

EDITH: I was also in love with Kenneth.

DREW: And you still are, aren't you?

EDITH: Is it possible to be in love with a memory?

DREW: Oh, yes, indeed.

EDITH: Is that your secret?

DREW: All right. If you must know...and your lips are sealed.

EDITH: My honor as a girl scout.

COME OUT, COME OUT, WHEREVER YOU ARE

DREW: I've been having an affair with Charlotte Pevny.

EDITH: You're not serious?

DREW: No, but I'm afraid she is.

EDITH: Does Herbert know?

DREW: Not so far. But things have been getting out of hand, and I've been trying to break it off.

EDITH: Serves you right. Seducing that sweet, dear child.

DREW: Sweet dear child? She practically raped me.

EDITH: Yes, of course. You're so attractive.

DREW: You used to think so, until Kenneth came along.

EDITH: I still think you're attractive.

DREW: Do you? Why do you shake your head?

EDITH: Why are men so needy? They claim to be the stronger sex, but they constantly have to be reassured. *(After a moment)* Brenda's become so possessive. She accuses me of flirting with everyone, male, female, animal, vegetable.

DREW: Has she any grounds for her suspicion?

EDITH: When I moved in, I never made any promises. She...and her friends...seem to have taken me for granted, and it's become oppressive. She wants to go to Germany this summer, and I'm not quite sure I want to go. It's funny, the things I found so attractive about her, her coolness, her efficiency, her no nonsense approach to life, they're just the things that...just turn me off. I think maybe we need some space. You have no such problem. You're free as the wind, officially.

DREW: I'm free of Charlotte, at any rate...as far as I'm concerned. What is it about me? I seem to be catnip for married women.

EDITH: It's your fatal charm.

DREW: I never tried to hook up with Charlotte. She was the one. And the one before that...

EDITH: Good Lord! How many were there?

DREW: Five. That includes the housekeeper who took my virginity back at the fraternity house at Yale.

EDITH: You're just a victim of female aggression.

DREW: As a matter of fact, Dr. Freud, that's the story of my life.

EDITH: Poor Drew. His fatal charm has been his undoing.

DREW: (After a moment) Has Brenda any reason to feel jealous?

EDITH: Any specific reason? No.

DREW: You're on the cusp, and she's aware of it. That's why she wants to whisk you away to Germany. Since you don't speak German, maybe you're safe there. And you can't make up your mind. Or maybe you have made up your mind, and you're afraid to admit it. Or maybe what you really are is a prisoner.

EDITH: A prisoner?

DREW: A prisoner of your memory.

COME OUT, COME OUT, WHEREVER YOU ARE

EDITH: No one can ever take Kenneth's place. I can't expect that. Oh, I wish I was seventy...eighty...and all this was behind me.

DREW: I'm not so sure that age is the answer.

EDITH: What is the answer?

DREW: Finding the right one.

EDITH: Kenneth was the right one, and he's gone. Then I thought Brenda might be the right one...and maybe she still is. Maybe I'm expecting too much from a relationship. What?

DREW: How about a game of tennis?

EDITH: Now?

DREW: No, you idiot! Tomorrow. Nine o'clock. Make it ten. How about it?

EDITH: I'm sort of rusty.

DREW: I'm no fool. You still have your racquet, don't you? The one I bought you for your graduation?

EDITH: It's probably upstairs somewhere.

DREW: If you can't find it, I've got an extra one.

EDITH: All right.

DREW: I've gotta go. I've had quite a day, and I am beat. Say good night for me, will you?

EDITH; Yes, of course.

COME OUT, COME OUT, WHEREVER YOU ARE

DREW: See you at ten.

> *(DREW kisses EDITH on the cheek, and starts off. As LILY enters with HAL, DREW returns, kisses EDITH on the lips and goes off.)*

LILY; Where is Drew off to?

EDITH: What? Oh. He asked me to say good night. He had a busy day. Do you remember that tennis racquet Drew gave me for my graduation?

LILY: What about it?

EDITH: Do I still have it?

LILY: If you do, it's in your room, and I never go poking about in your room. What I mean to say is, it's still your room.

> *(EDITH goes off.)*

LILY: *(SHE looks at HAL.)* What?

HAL: I didn't say anything.

LILY: I'm not as silly as some people think I am. When can I have my stand?

HAL: I'll get right to it. Good night, Mrs. Byington. And thank you for the dinner.

LILY: What's that? Yes, yes, dear. Thank you.

> *(HAL hesitates then goes off. LILY stands deep in thought, then smiles, very pleased with herself, as the lights come down.)*

ACT TWO

Scene One

(Afternoon, the following day. The doorbell rings. After a moment it rings again. HAL, in working clothes enters and looks around. MARIAN, in uniform, carrying a dust cloth enters.)

MARIAN: What are you doing here?

HAL: I've come to see Mrs. Byington. I've got the plans for her plant stand. Is she here?

MARIAN: That's a good question.

HAL: I'll just leave them here then. Tell her to give me a call. My place, by the way could use a cleaning.

MARIAN: I'm kinda busy. Monday, maybe, around nine o'clock.

HAL: Okay.

MARIAN: Incidentally, what are you gonna do about that boy of yours?

HAL: What do you mean?

MARIAN: Did you know that Billy stole a cell phone from the hardware store? He tried to, at any rate.

HAL: When was this?

MARIAN: Just the other day.

HAL: Joe never said anything to me about it.

COME OUT, COME OUT, WHEREVER YOU ARE

MARIAN: That's because Billy started to cry and swore he'd never do it again.

HAL: I guess I'd better sit down and have a talk with that boy.

MARIAN: I know you got a rough deal, Hal, ..but I think it's about time you went out and found yourself a wife. I think that that's what Betsy would have wanted, don't you?

HAL: Is that a proposal?

MARIAN: I'm serious. That boy needs a mother.

(LILY enters.)

LILY: Marian? Oh, Hal, dear. Good morning.

HAL: Good morning. I've got those plans for your plant stand.

LILY: That was quick.

HAL: There you are. *(HE hands her the plans.)*

LILY: Oh, you're such a clever man. *(To MARIAN)* Are you through in here?

MARIAN: I haven't started.

LILY: Then you can start here later. I want you to straighten up Edith's room first. It's a mess.

MARIAN: What's the rush? She doesn't live here anymore.

LILY: Do I have to explain to you why I want things done?

COME OUT, COME OUT, WHEREVER YOU ARE

MARIAN: It helps sometimes, when what you want done doesn't make any sense.

> (*MARIAN goes off, muttering under her breath as JOSHUA enters.*)

JOSHUA: What's the matter with Marian?

LILY: That woman will be the death of me.

JOSHUA: Why don't you fire her?

LILY: Don't be ridiculous. When can I have my plant stand?

HAL: Tuesday all right?

LILY: Tuesday's fine. As a matter of fact, I make perfect sense. (*SHE goes off.*)

JOSHUA: Have you ever made a speech?

HAL: No, sir.

JOSHUA: Why I've been chosen to address the graduating class, I'll never know. I know a little something about English literature, that's about all I know. What do you say to young people when they have to face a world that's as messy as ours is today, wars, poverty, massacres, rape? I need a drink. How about a glass of Bailey's Irish Cream?

HAL: Okay.

JOSHUA: (*HE pours two glasses of wine.*) That's what I like about you, Hal. You take life as it comes.

COME OUT, COME OUT, WHEREVER YOU ARE

HAL: I never aimed very high, Professor. And there are times when I regret it.

(JOSHUA hands HAL his wine.)

HAL: Thank you. *(HE sips his wine.)* Do you think it's too late for me to get an education?

JOSHUA: What sort of an education?

HAL: Well, there's a lot that I don't know.

JOSHUA: *(HE laughs.)* Is there really? What's troubling you, Son?

HAL: Well, Billy, for one. Sometimes he does get out of hand.

JOSHUA: In raising a child, I'd say common sense is what's required. And I'd give you an A for common sense. You read a lot, don't you?

HAL: Whenever I have time.

JOSHUA: What do you read?

HAL: Biography, history. I guess it all depends on what I'm curious about.

JOSHUA: Then I'd say you're getting the best education that's available.

HAL: If you don't mind my asking, how are Edith and Miss Lewis getting along? You see, when Kenny left he asked me to sort of keep an eye on Edith.

JOSHUA: Did he now? Well, frankly, I think that relationship is about to be cancelled.

COME OUT, COME OUT, WHEREVER YOU ARE

HAL: Oh?

JOSHUA: You thinking about calling on Edith, by any chance?

HAL: I don't think Edith would wanna be tied down to a widower with a son, and no education to speak of.

JOSHUA: As a matter of fact I always thought that you two had a lot in common. Down to earth and unpretentious, amazingly enough, when you think of the mother she comes from.

HAL: Don't you think that Edith has more in common with someone like...Drew Timmons, for example?

JOSHUA: Heaven forbid.

(EDITH and DREW enter dressed for tennis.)

EDITH & DREW: Good morning.

JOSHUA: Morning? It's way past noon.

DREW: Good noon.

JOSHUA: What are you two so chipper about?

DREW: Shall you tell them, or shall I? Edith, fool that she is, has consented to be my wife. Well? Isn't anybody going to say something...like congratulations, best of luck?

HAL: Congratulations.

EDITH: Thank you

DREW: Not a word from my father-in-law to be?

COME OUT, COME OUT, WHEREVER YOU ARE

HAL: Well, I've got some work to do. *(HE shakes hands with DREW.)* Best of luck. *(HE approaches EDITH.)* I'm very happy for you. *(He is about to shake her hand but, impulsively, HE kisses her on her on the cheek and goes off.)*

DREW: What an odd fellow that man is.

EDITH: He's a lovely man. He ought to have someone. I'm going to take a quick shower. Drew and I are going for a drive, and find a nice quiet place for dinner. Daddy?

JOSHUA: Yes, dear?

EDITH: Nothing. *(SHE goes off.)*

JOSHUA: Kind of sudden, isn't it?

DREW: No one's more surprised than I am.

JOSHUA: Are you quite sure you know what you're doing?

DREW: I know, I know. But I think it's time I settled down.

JOSHUA: That girl's been through a lot, Drew.

DREW: I'm aware of that, and I'm aware of your skepticism.

JOSHUA: You haven't set a date, have you?

DREW: We would like to spend our honeymoon in Paris, this summer, which doesn't give us very much time, does it?.

JOSHUA: I see.

DREW: Edith wants a small wedding, right here, in the house...as

31

soon as possible. Now, Joshua, don't look so stern. I'm really not a scoundrel. I'll make you a fine son-in-law.

JOSHUA: What brought this on, may I ask?

DREW: I've always had my eye on Edith. As a matter of fact, before Ken came along, I thought seriously about her.

JOSHUA: Ken's been gone for almost three years.

DREW: I'm aware of that.

JOSHUA: So what's been stopping you?

DREW: You know perfectly well what I've been up to.

JOSHUA: That's what worries me.

DREW: I've been branded. Is that it? The scarlet letter? I'm growing up, Josh. Give me a break.

JOSHUA: Don't you think you ought to take a little time to think things through? Marriage, Drew...it's a big step, you know.

DREW: Is it really?

JOSHUA: And Edith leads with her heart.

DREW: And so, for that matter, do I.

JOSHUA: Well, frankly, Drew, I'm not so sure you have a heart.

DREW: Joshua, what a cruel thing to say.

JOSHUA: I'm sorry. It's just that marriage, in order to work, has got to involve two temperaments that are compatible.

COME OUT, COME OUT, WHEREVER YOU ARE

DREW: And you think that the two of us...

JOSHUA: Are not in the same ball park. That's not to say that I don't like you, Drew. I'm fond of you. I enjoy your company. You know that. I just wish you'd take more time to think things through.

(MARIAN enters.)

MARIAN: *(To JOSHUA)* The missus would like a word with you.

JOSHUA: Oh, oh. Excuse me. *(HE goes off.)*

MARIAN: What do you think you're doing?

DREW: Not you, too.

MARIAN: Edith is a fine woman, Professor.

DREW: I'm aware of that.

MARIAN: Don't you think she's been through enough already?

DREW: You know, it's strange the way people think they have the right to stand in judgement. Just because I've lived a full life, trod where others feared to tread...

MARIAN: Don't you start getting fancy with me, 'cause I know you Drew Timmons. As a matter of fact, I know you better than you know yourself.

DREW: Do you really? Well, I'd appreciate it if you'd stick to what concerns you.

MARIAN: Edith happens to concern me. I've known her since she was a little girl. And my nephew concerns me too. And, it might interest you to know, he's lost his job in the mail room.

COME OUT, COME OUT, WHEREVER YOU ARE

DREW: I'm sorry to hear that.

MARIAN: Why don't you to give him a call. I'm really worried about him.

DREW: Your nephew, dear Marian, is a confused young man with a drinking problem, and I've done what I can for the boy.

MARIAN: He's not a boy, and you must have given him a reason to take you seriously.

DREW: That young man's your nephew, Marian, and he's your responsibility, not mine.

MARIAN: Does Edith know about you and Roger?

DREW: My relationship with Roger has nothing to do with my relationship with my future wife.

(EDITH enters, dressed for the afternoon.)

EDITH: Is there anything wrong?

MARIAN: I think Mr. Timmons might have something to talk to you about. *(SHE goes off.)*

EDITH: Drew?

DREW: Do you have any regrets?

EDITH: About what?

DREW: About your life? About the decisions you've made?

EDITH: Offhand, I can't think of any.

COME OUT, COME OUT, WHEREVER YOU ARE

DREW: What about Brenda?

EDITH: No, I don't regret our relationship. I needed her. She needed me. Neither of us made any promises.

DREW: And yet there may be people standing in judgement. What are you? Who are you?

EDITH: I'm an associate professor, and I'm a woman.

DREW: In love with another woman?

EDITH: I guess. But maybe love isn't the answer...the entire answer, that is.

DREW: Compatibility, according to your father.

EDITH: Why, yes. I think that's as good a word as any.

DREW: Do you think we're compatible?

EDITH: I wouldn't be willing to marry you if I didn't think we have enough in common to make each other happy. What's this all about?

DREW: As you know, I haven't been exactly celibate. There was this affair with Charlotte Pevney.

EDITH: Is that what you two were discussing?

DREW: I really resent Marian's interference.

EDITH: Im sure she means well.

DREW: She's concerned about her nephew. Roger happens to be

a very confused young man, with a drinking problem. I felt sorry for the boy, and I went out of my way to get him a job in the University mail room, and now the young man thinks he's in love with me.

EDITH: Have you given him any encouragement?

DREW: I've made no promises. It's just one of those boyhood infatuations, and I'm sure he'll get over it eventually.

MARIAN: I see.

DREW: I'd better change, if we're going for a drive. We are going for a drive, aren't we?

EDITH: Yes. Yes, of course.

DREW: See you in an hour.

    (HE kisses her and goes off. EDITH stands lost in thought. After a moment, LILY enters.)

LILY: Well, we've got to get to work. We'll have the ceremony outside, in the garden. It's such a lovely time of the year. Come along. We've got to sit down and make a list. *(SHE starts off, stops and turns.)* Are you all right?

EDITH: Yes. Yes, I'm fine.

LILY: Come along then.

    (LILY links her arm in EDITH's and leads her off as the lights come down.)

Scene Two

(One month later. Sunday noon, a beautiful summer day. Music and the low murmur of voices are heard from offstage. DREW. dressed in tails is pacing nervously. MARIAN, dressed for the wedding, enters hurriedly from the outside.)

DREW: Are we ready to start?

(MARIAN stands, collecting herself.)

DREW: What is it? What's the matter?

MARIAN: *(SHE hands him a note.)* Read this.

DREW: What is it?

MARIAN: I've just come from the hospital. Read the damn thing.

(DREW reads the note.)

MARIAN: He swallowed a bunch of pills. He called me a little while ago, to say good-bye. I rushed over to his room. By time I got there, he was half conscious. I called emergency, and they sent an ambulance, and now they're pumping his stomach.

DREW: Do they think he'll pull through?

MARIAN: And what if he does? What's to stop him from trying it again? I warned you, Professor.

DREW: Where is he now?

MARIAN: I just told you. He's in the hospital!! He's in the emergency room.

DREW: All right, all right. What do you want me to do?

COME OUT, COME OUT, WHEREVER YOU ARE

MARIAN: You do what your conscience tells you to do.

DREW: I'm getting married in a couple of minutes.

MARIAN: I hope you'll be happy, Professor. *(SHE starts off.)*

DREW: Marian...

MARIAN: What?

DREW: I'm fond of the boy, I really am.

MARIAN: Yes, I know you are. And you did all you could for him, didn't you?

DREW: You really think he'll try it again?

MARIAN: Why don't you ask him yourself?

DREW: I can't leave now. *(After a moment)* I might be able to run over for just a second...just to make sure he's all right...but I don't have my car.

MARIAN: My car's nearby.

DREW: I should leave word.

MARIAN: I'll take care of it.

DREW: All right. Let's go.

> *(DREW leaves, followed by MARIAN. A moment later JOSHUA and HAL enter, dressed for the wedding. HAL looks around.)*

JOSHUA: What's the matter?

COME OUT, COME OUT, WHEREVER YOU ARE

HAL: I thought I saw Drew come in here a moment ago.

JOSHUA: He must have stepped out for some air. You're not nervous, are you?

HAL: I've never been a best man before.

JOSHUA: You've got the ring, haven't you?

HAL: *(HE pats his jacket pocket.)* Right here.

JOSHUA: That's all you have to worry about.

HAL: If you say so.

JOSHUA: What you need is a drink. What can I get you? And don't ask me for a coke. What kind of an Irishman are you?

HAL: What are you gonna have?

JOSHUA: A Scotch, straight up.

HAL: I'll have the same.

> *(JOSHUA pours two drinks and hands one to HAL.)*

JOSHUA: To weddings. They're a blessing and a curse.

HAL: For better or for worse

JOSHUA Here, here.

> *(THEY drink.)*

JOSHUA: Do you remember your wedding day?

COME OUT, COME OUT, WHEREVER YOU ARE

HAL: As if it was yesterday. Betsy was always a pretty woman but, that day, she was beautiful. And she looked so fragile, as if she might break, if you held her too tight.

JOSHUA: Lily and I eloped.

HAL: Did you really?

JOSHUA: Her father did not approve of me. They were Boston royalty, and I was just a poor kid from the. other side of the tracks. It took a year or two before they came around. Her father, that is. He was an arrogant son-of-a-bitch.

HAL: *(After a moment)* You don't approve of Drew, do you?

JOSHUA: As a son-in-law, no. But actually, I'm rather fond of Drew. He's a charming man, but he's got a lot of growing up to do.

(MARIAN enters.)

JOSHUA: So there you are. Lily's been looking all over for you.

MARIAN: I was over at the hospital.

JOSHUA: The hospital?

MARIAN: My nephew had an accident.

JOSHUA: I'm sorry to hear that. Is he all right?

MARIAN: I think he'll pull through.

JOSHUA: You haven't seen Drew, by an chance?

COME OUT, COME OUT, WHEREVER YOU ARE

MARIAN: Drew's over at the hospital.

JOSHUA: What's he doing at the hospital?

MARIAN: He's concerned about my nephew?

JOSHUA: This is a fine time to visit someone at the hospital.

(LILY enters dressed for the wedding.)

LILY: Where have you been?

MARIAN: My nephew had an accident. He's at the hospital.

LILY: Oh, I'm so sorry. Is he all right?

MARIAN: They think he'll pull through.

LILY: Oh, I'm so glad. Has anyone seen Drew?

JOSHUA: Drew's at the hospital.

LILY: Drew too?!

JOSHUA: He's visiting Marian's nephew.

LILY: You're not serious.

MARIAN: They were sort of close.

LILY: Close? What do you mean, "close"?

JOSHUA: That's a good question.

LILY: Marian?

COME OUT, COME OUT, WHEREVER YOU ARE

MARIAN: I think the professor's the only one that can answer that.

LILY: We're almost ready to start. Judge Harper's arrived, and he has another wedding to go to after this. What am I supposed to tell people?. What sort of an accident was your nephew in?

MARIAN: He swallowed some pills.

LILY: What kind of pills?

JOSHUA: What difference does it make?

LILY: Well, I must say, for a grown man, Drew's behaving very oddly.

JOSHUA: No comment.

LILY: I wouldn't blame Edith, if she called the whole thing off. Either way... This is impossible.

(EDITH enters in her wedding dress.)

LILY: Drew's in the hospital, visiting a sick friend. Ask Marian.

MARIAN: My nephew, Roger, had an accident.

EDITH: Oh, I'm so sorry.

MARIAN: I think he'll be all right. He swallowed some pills.

EDITH: I see.

LILY: This is unspeakable. What shall I tell people?

COME OUT, COME OUT, WHEREVER YOU ARE

EDITH: Tell them there's been an emergency, and to please be patient.

LILYU: And when they ask questions, what am I supposed to say?

EDITH: Think Billie Burke.

LILY: Really, Edith, this is not the movies. Come along, Joshua. I'm not going to face those people all by myself. And, Marian, will you please get on the phone and talk to Drew?

MARIAN: What would you like me to tell him?

LILY: Tell him to stop acting like an idiot.

(MARIAN goes off.)

LILY: Joshua?

JOSHUA: Coming, dear.

(JOSHUA follows LILY off.)

EDITH: I feel kind of foolish, to say the least. What are you smiling at?

HAL: I was just wondering what Kenny would have said at a time like this? He had a great sense of humor.

EDITH: That's one of the reasons I fell in love with him. I haven't had much luck, have I?

HAL: Incidentally...

EDITH: What?

COME OUT, COME OUT, WHEREVER YOU ARE

HAL: This may not be the proper time, but you remember that snapshot I spoke about...the one with me and Kenny?

EDITH: What about it?

HAL: I kept meaning to drop it off, but this time I remembered, and I brought it along.

EDITH: May I see it?

(HE takes out the snapshot and hands it to her.)

EDITH: He looks so young. You both look so young.

HAL: We must have been about sixteen or so.

EDITH: May I keep this?

HAL: I brought it for you.

EDITH: Thank you. *(SHE places the picture on a shelf, so that it's easily visible.)*

HAL: I never told you this. But, when Kenny left for the army, he said to me, "Hal, I want you to keep an eye on Edie for me." and I said I would. And I guess haven't done a very good job, have I?

EDITH: You've had problems of your own.

HAL: I think one of the reasons he turned to me, aside from the fact, that we were good friends. Well, the fact of the matter is, he knew that I did have a sort of crush on you.

EDITH: Did you really?

COME OUT, COME OUT, WHEREVER YOU ARE

HAL: Of course, we really don't have that much in common do we, you being a professor and all that...

EDITH: Assistant professor.

HAL: Assistant professor. I'm not really that well educated,

EDITH: You think a degree makes you any the wiser? And, as a matter of fact...I always thought...you were kind of cute.

HAL: Cute?

EDITH: Attractive.

HAL: Did you really?

EDITH: There were lots of girls that thought you were...attractive. And I'm sure you were aware of it.

HAL: I never thought I was ugly. Incidentally, I never did thank you, for arranging for Billy to take that aptitude test.

EDITH: I think he's a fine boy, Hal.

HAL: Well, he's sure a handful. I can tell you that. Anyway, I want you to know, that if I can ever help you in any way, any way at all, you can count on me.

EDITH: Thank you.

(DREW enters.)

DREW: I'm sorry.

HAL: I'd better let people know you're here. Excuse me. *(HE goes off.)*

45

COME OUT, COME OUT, WHEREVER YOU ARE

DREW: I'm sorry.

EDITH: You said that.

DREW: I need a drink. *(HE pours a drink and downs it.)* I can't go through with it, Edith. I feel awful, I really do. But I think it'd be worse, if I were to go ahead and marry you.

EDITH: Are you in love with Roger?

DREW: Love? I don't know if you'd call it love? I mean, what is love really? He needs me, and I've come to realize, even though I've been afraid to admit it...I need him, as well. I've gone for all these years, fighting what was inside of me, going from one affair to the other, as a refuge, I guess. And then when that young man came along... It was pity, at first. We met in a bar, a gay bar, and he was drunk.

EDITH: I see.

DREW: Roger has a drinking problem. I wanted to nurse him, I wanted to take care of him. I wanted him to want me, too, but I fought it. I fought it continually, and, at the same time, I kept reaching out to him. Finally, he became dependent on me, the way I wanted him to, and that's when I turned away. I was frightened. Did I want to spend the rest of my life with this damaged young man, who was twelve years younger than I was?

EDITH: And do you?

DREW: God help me. Edith, I do. I really do. Can you forgive me?

EDITH: There's nothing to forgive.

DREW: And here I've put you in this embarrassing position.

COME OUT, COME OUT, WHEREVER YOU ARE

EDITH: Like you said, there's no point in our being miserable for the rest of our lives.

DREW: Would you like me to go out and make an announcement?

EDITH: I'll take care of it.

DREW: You sure?

EDITH: I'm positive. Go. *(SHE takes hold of him by the shoulders, and faces him toward the doorway.)* Go. *(SHE gives him a shove.)*

DREW: *(HE turns and kisses her.)* Thank you. And good luck.

(DREW goes off as LILY and JOSHUA reenter.)

LILY: Where is he going?

EDITH: Back to the hospital.

LILY: Will you please tell me what is going on?

EDITH: Will you please ask Hal to come in?

LILY: I asked you a question.

EDITH: And I asked you to send in Hal. I'd like to speak to him...alone.

JOSHUA: I think we'd better do as Edith says.

LILY: I think the world's gone mad. *(SHE goes off.)*

JOSHUA: Good luck.

(JOSHUA goes off. HAL reenters.)

COME OUT, COME OUT, WHEREVER YOU ARE

HAL: You wanted to see me. Where's Drew?

EDITH: He's gone.

HAL: Oh?.

EDITH: Would you like to marry me?

HAL: Yes. Now?

EDITH: Now's as good a time as any. We're not getting any younger and, since people are out there waiting for someone to get married.

HAL: Are you sure you want to do this?

EDITH: I am, if you are.

HAL: Most certainly am, if you are.

EDITH: Then it's settled.

HAL: What about a license?

EDITH: Since Judge Harper's performing the ceremony, I'm sure it'll be no problem. Have you got the ring?

HAL: Right here.

EDITH: Would you bring in my parents, please?

HAL: Yes, of course.

> (*HAL goes off. EDITH stands waiting. SHE looks at the snapshot then straightens it. LILY and JOSHUA enter, followed by HAL.*)

48

COME OUT, COME OUT, WHEREVER YOU ARE

LILY: Yes. Well?

EDITH: Hal and I have decided...

HAL: I'm going to take Drew's place.

EDITH: We're getting married.

(THEY look at one another, and THEY kiss.)

LILY: Well... I guess you both know what you're doing. And at this point...frankly, my dears, I don't...

JOSHUA: Give a damn. Yes, I know. Congratulations. *(HE kisses EDITH and embraces HAL.)*

LILY: I'll tell everyone to take their places. *(SHE starts off, then stops.)*

EDITH: Yes, Mother, what is it?

LILY: I'm trying to think. Was it It Happened One Night or The Philadelphia Story?

JOSHUA: What on earth are you talking about?

LILY: It'll come to me. *(SHE goes off.)*

(There's a moment of silence offstage, then wedding music is heard. LILY reenters. A wedding march is heard.)

JOSHUA: That's you, Son. Just walk straight down the aisle, and stand in front of the judge.

(HAL stands erect, squares his shoulders and walks slowly off.)

49

COME OUT, COME OUT WHEREVER YOU ARE

LILY: He does have a certain dignity, doesn't he?

EDITH: He always did have.

> *(The bridal entrance music is heard. LILY and JOSHUA link arms with EDITH. THEY start slowly off. LILY stops.)*

LILY: The Philadelphia Story.

JOSHUA: What about it?

LILY: The ending. *(After a moment)* At least I think it was.

> *(The lights come down as THEY go off.)*

LOVE AMONG THE ARTISTS
A Bi-Sexual Comedy

CAST OF CHARACTERS

Pamela Buford

Brian Hastings

Gertie Myers

Keith Garrick

Kay Charles Garrick

SCENE
Living room.
The Garrick summer home in New England

ACT ONE

Scene One

(The living room of the Garrick summer home. The doorbell rings. A long pause. The doorbell rings again. Another long pause. PAMELA BUFORD and BRIAN HASTINGS, both in their mid-twenties, enter rather tentatively.)

BRIAN: There's no one home.

PAM: A brilliant deduction.

BRIAN: Let's go.

(PAM walks about inspecting the room.)

BRIAN: Pam!

(PAM sits in an easy chair, takes a filter-tipped cigar from her purse and lights it.)

BRIAN: You are out of your mind!

PAM: What are you, a man or a mouse?

BRIAN: You know perfectly well what I am.

PAM: It's them. This room. It's them. *(As Petruchio in "Taming of the Shrew:")* "Good morrow, Kate; for that's your name I hear. *(As Katherine)* "Well have you heard, but something hard of hearing. They call me Katherine that do talk of me." *(As Petruchio)* You lie, in faith: for you are called plain Kate, And bonny Kate and sometimes Kate the curst; but Kate, the prettiest Kate in Christendom."

BRIAN: I'm leaving.

LOVE AMONG THE ARTISTS

PAM: Stay! Put one foot across that threshold and I shall break this vase.

BRIAN: My God! That's a genuine antique. Put it down! I'm staying, I'm staying.

PAM: We were invited here...for tea.

BRIAN: So you said. Please, be careful with that vase.

PAM: *(After replacing the vase she produces a note.)* What does that say?

BRIAN: *(Reading)* "My dear Miss Buford..." It says nothing about bringing a friend.

PAM: An invitation always includes a companion, And besides, I didn't trust my self, alone with Keith Garrick.

BRIAN: Keith Garrick is a happily married man.

PAM: My dear child, you are so naive.

BRIAN: And we do have a rehearsal at four, you know. And will you please stop touching things. And Pam, you are dropping ashes all over the rug. Where are you going?

PAM: Maybe he's out on the terrace.

BRIAN: I am leaving. Good-bye.

> *(PAM sets down her cigar on an ash tray and falls to the floor.)*

PAM: Ohhh.

LOVE AMONG THE ARTISTS

BRIAN: Pam?! Get up!

PAM: Where am I?

> *(BRIAN starts off as GERTIE MYERS, a woman in her seventies, enters from the terrace, unseen by the two young people.)*

PAM: Brian, don't leave me. I'm pregnant.

GERTIE: Good Lord! You young people nowadays. I'm Gertie Myers. How do you do. *(SHE shakes hands with PAM on the floor and then with BRIAN.)* I'm so glad you could come.

BRIAN: Thank you. Pamela, will you please get up. She's not really pregnant you know.

GERTIE: What is that awful smell? Do you smoke cigars, young man?

BRIAN: Not me.

GERTIE: My God! It's still alive. Put it out, my dear. Put it out. No, no, no. Not in that. Use that one over there. Have you been here long?

PAM: Not really, no.

BRIAN: We just arrived.

GERTIE: I was in the garden tending to the petunias. I'm British, you know. I thought we might have our tea out on the terrace, but it's a little chilly out there, so I think we'll have tea in here.

PAM: Will Mr. Garrick be joining us?

LOVE AMONG THE ARTISTS

GERTIE: I'm not quite sure. *(SHE goes off.)*

BRIAN Who is she?

PAM: It's Gertie Myers. She was a star, years ago. She and her sister, Lily had this act. They were quite famous.

BRIAN: Keith Garrick may not even be here. As a matter of fact, he's probably in London right now.

(GERTIE reenters.)

GERTIE: You're going to meet him, I promise you. The water's heating. *(SHE goes off.)*

PAM: So there you are. And you know perfectly well that you're just as excited as I am.

BRIAN: Yes...well...he is sexy. But I don't think he was really there, at our performance.

PAM: The note was signed by him.

BRIAN: Not necessarily. Maybe she was the one that signed it, and she's obviously a little ditsy.

(GERTIE reenters with the tea tray.)

GERTIE: When you reach seventy five, if you reach seventy five, my dear, you may be a little ditsy, too.

BRIAN: I didn't mean. Actually....you're really quite charming.

GERTIE: Hmmmmmm. *(Addressing PAM)* Lemon or milk?

PAM: Lemon, thank you.

LOVE AMONG THE ARTISTS

GERTIE: One lump or two?

PAM: Two, thank you?

GERTIE: And you?

BRIAN: Milk, thank you.

GERTIE: At least you're civilized.

BRIAN: One lump.

(GERTIE hands BRIAN his tea. The phone rings.)

GERTIE: Excuse me. *(SHE picks up the phone.)* Hello. Yes, Lily, I'm perfectly fine. I'm entertaining some guests at the moment. I'll call you back. I said I would call you back. *(SHE hangs up.)* That was my sister. I was the talented one. She was the pretty one, and now she's a widow...Sir Henry died last year, you know, and now that she's all alone, she suddenly remembers that she's my devoted sibling.

PAM: She lives in London, doesn't she?

GERTIE: Very comfortably, I might add. Where were we? Oh, do have some biscuits. They're very good.

(The doorbell rings.)

GERTIE: Oh, dear! Excuse me. *(SHE goes off.)*

BRIAN: I don't think we ought to stay very long.

PAM: I'm going to stay until I meet him.

LOVE AMONG THE ARTISTS

BRIAN: Well, if he's not here by three thirty, I am leaving...for our rehearsal.

(GERTIE reenters with a letter.)

GERTIE: *(SHE eyes the letter suspiciously.)* Special delivery letters are always rather frightening, don't you think? It's for Keith. I'm so tempted. It's from the Royal Shakespeare Company.

PAM: He's scheduled to do Hamlet there, isn't he?

GERTIE: Yes. He's been dreaming about it for years. Get thee behind me. *(SHE places the letter conspicuously on a table.)* How's the tea?

PAM: It's fine.

BRIAN: Did Mr. Garrick actually come to see our production of Barefoot In The Park?

GERTIE: He most certainly did. And we thought you were both charming.

PAM: Did Miss Charles come as well?

GERTIE: No, dear. She's recovering from...a procedure. As a matter of fact, she's due back home very shortly. Keith has gone to fetch her. Do have some more tea, dear.

PAM: *(SHE lifts her cup and it tips over.)* Damn.

BRIAN: Honestly!

PAM: Oh, shut up!

LOVE AMONG THE ARTISTS

GERTIE: And that's such a pretty frock. Cold water...at once. There's a bathroom at the head of the stairs. Go...quickly.

(PAM goes off.)

BRIAN: You're staring at me.

GERTIE: It's remarkable.

BRIAN: What?

GERTIE: You are the spitting image of Michael, my dear, dead husband. Come with me.

BRIAN: Where are we going?

GERTIE: I want to show you a photograph. You needn't worry, dear. I'm not going to try and seduce you.

BRIAN: It wouldn't do you any good. I'm gay.

GERTIE: Well, of course you are.

> *(THEY go off. KAY CHARLES GARRICK, a striking looking woman in her early forties, enters. SHE sighs, looks about the room and runs her fingers over the furniture, testing for dust. KEITH GARRICK, a handsome man in his early forties enters. HE sets down the suitcase he's carrying, places his arms around KAY and kisses her.)*

KEITH: It's so good to have you back.

KAY: It's so good to be back. It looks like Gertie's entertaining.

KEITH: I asked her not to.

LOVE AMONG THE ARTISTS

KAY: Who is it? Do you know?

KEITH: It's a couple of actors from the Playhouse. With the kids in camp, and you in the hospital she's sort of lost.

KAY: You look so vigorous, and so healthy.

KEITH: And so will you, after we fatten you up. Well, you have lost some weight, and we're going to put some color into those lovely cheeks of yours; fill you with fresh country air and lots of sunshine.

KAY: And decent food. The food at that place was awful.

(KEITH sees the letter on the table and picks it up.)

KAY: What is it?

KEITH: A special delivery...from the Royal Shakespeare. Uh, oh! *(HE opens the letter and reads it.)*

KAY: What is it?

KEITH: I won't be doing Hamlet.

KAY: Oh, no!

KEITH: They want me to do...Othello!!

KAY: Othello?

KEITH: Barry Jefferson will be doing Hamlet, and I'll be doing Othello, without any makeup. Can you believe it?

KAY: Barry Jefferson is...

KEITH: Black. "The world is changing, Keith. We've got to keep up with the times. Color is now a non-issue." Hamlet is going to be black...

KAY: And Othello is going to be white. It doesn't make any sense. Unless, of course, they're going to rewrite Shakespeare. I mean they do refer to the color of his skin. It's in the script.

KEITH: I was hired to do Hamlet, and Hamlet is what I'm going to do.

KAY: Was it in your contract?

> (*KEITH goes off. KAY picks up the letter and reads it. PAMELA enters.*)

PAMELA: Oh!

KAY: Hello.

PAM: Hello, Miss Charles.

KAY: You must be...

PAM: I'm Pamela Buford. I'm an actress at the theatre.

KAY: Yes, of course, you are. Keith spoke about you, and he said you're very good.

> (*GERTIE reenters with BRIAN.*)

GERTIE: You're back! Oh, my dear, welcome home. (*SHE embraces her.*) Have you lost weight?

KAY: A little.

LOVE AMONG THE ARTISTS

(KEITH reenters, holding a contract.)

KEITH: That son-of-a-bitch!

GERTIE: What's wrong now?

KEITH: I'll be playing Othello.

GERTIE: Nonsense! You did sign a contract, didn't you?

KEITH: It just gives the dates. Hello, Brian. Hello, Pamela.

BRIAN: Hello.

PÁM: Hello.

KEITH: I'm sorry I never got backstage. We've got two kids in camp, and there's always an emergency. *(To KAY.)* This is ridiculous! Without even consulting me.

(The telephone rings.)

GERTIE: I'll get it. *(SHE picks up the phone.)* Hello. Who's calling? *(To KEITH)* It's the camp.

KAY: Is there anything wrong?

KEITH: *(HE takes the phone.)* Hello. This is Mr. Garrick. *(HE sighs.)* I'll be right over. *(HE hangs up.)*

KAY: What is it?

KEITH: It's Emily. She wants to come home. We've got to go out there and pick her up.

KAY: We will do nothing of the sort. She pestered us all year long about going to camp.

BRIAN: *(To Pam)* I think we ought to be going.

KEITH: I'm sorry. You'll come back, of course, the two of you. Gertie, you arrange it.

PAM: It's been nice meeting you both.

BRIAN: And you were wonderful, Miss Charles, in Taming Of The Shrew.

KAY: Why thank you, dear. You must come back soon.

BRIAN: Thank you.

PAM: Good-bye.

> *(PAM and BRIAN go off.)*

KAY: Oh, to be young again.

KEITH: Yes, old lady.

GERTIE: Are you going to pick up that child, or are you not?

KAY: He is not.

KEITH: Oh yes, he is.

KAY: And what about Tony? Are you going to pick him up too?

KEITH: Tony's a man.

KAY: A man?

LOVE AMONG THE ARTISTS

KEITH: He's verging on puberty. *(To GERTIE)* Oh, by the way. Lily called before I left. I forgot to tell you.

KAY: She is your sister, Gertie.

GERTIE: When the mood strikes her.

KAY: She's lonely.

GERTIE: Oh, go look after your offsprings.

KEITH: Are you coming with me?

KAY: Yes, of course I'm coming with you. *(To GERTIE)* We'll probably have dinner at the inn. If we do, we'll call you and you can join us.

> *(KEITH and KAY go off. GERTIE picks up the phone and dials.)*

GERTIE: Is this the infamous Lady Hawthorne? Now look here, Lily. I did not say I would call you right back. What's that? Well, Keith just told me, Of course, I care about you, dear. You're my only living relative, the last leaf on the tree, so to speak.

> *(The lights come down.)*

Scene Two

(Late that evening. GERTIE is on the sofa. SHE's nodded off, a book in her lap. KAY and KEITH enter from the outside. Seeing GERTIE asleep, THEY start off quietly, hand in hand.)

GERTIE: *(Looking up)* Why are you creeping about like that? Where are the children?

KAY: They're at the camp.

GERTIE: I thought you were bringing them home.

KAY: Whatever gave you that idea?

GERTIE: How is Emily?

KAY: Emily's perfectly fine.

KEITH: And Tony's won a trophy...in archery.

GERTIE: Is that what they do out there, shoot bows and arrows?

KEITH: *(HE picks up the book on Gertie's lap.)* You're really not right for Desdemona, you know.

GERTIE: All that fuss over a handkerchief.

KEITH: *(To KAY)* You must be tired.

KAY: I could use a drink.

KEITH: Are you allowed?

KAY: My digestive system's perfectly fine. Pour me some brandy.

GERTIE: Pour me one, too.

LOVE AMONG THE ARTISTS

(KEITH pours three brandies. HE hands one to KAY.)

KAY: Thank you, dear.

(KEITH hands a brandy to GERTIE.)

GERTIE: To Othello.

KEITH: Must you remind me?

(THEY drink.)

GERTIE: I was thinking...

KEITH: Uh oh!

GERTIE: The season at the Playhouse ends in two weeks, and the theatre is dark. Why don't you do Othello there, and invite the powers that be? When they see an Othello in white face, they might just come to their senses. And I'm sure Mr. Papadopolous would be delighted. He's been after you for years to do a show at the Playhouse.

KAY: I think that's a splendid idea,

KEITH: Would you be up to doing Desdemona?

KAY: No.

GERTIE: What about Emilia?

KAY: Emilia?!

GERTIE: It is a supporting role... Of course...

KAY: There are no small roles.

LOVE AMONG THE ARTISTS

GERTIE: Only small actors.

KAY: *(SHE shrugs.)* If you really want to go ahead with it.

KEITH: I'm curious. What sort of a response would there be to a white Othello? I mean...really! What time is it? *(HE checks his watch.)* Papadopolous is usually at the theatre till, at least, eleven. Do we have the number?

GERTIE: It's right there, in our little black book.

KEITH: *(HE consults the pad next to the phone and dials.)* Hello? Dmitri, it's Keith. I was wondering. You're dark in three weeks, and I'd be interested in trying out Othello for a week. *(HE places his hand on the mouth of the phone and turns to GERTIE and KAY.)* He's delighted. *(Back on the phone)* And perhaps we can persuade some of your resident company to stay on. Let's talk in the morning. Say ten, ten-thirty? Oh, she's fine. Thank you. I most certainly will. Thank you, Dmitri. *(HE hangs up.)* Dmitri sends you his best.

   (The doorbell rings.)

KEITH: Who could that be, at this hour?

GERTIE: It's probably the children.

KEITH: Children? What children?

GERTIE: Pam and Brian. I invited them over for a drink. You said to have them back. I'll get the door.

KEITH: Relax. I'll get the door.

   (KEITH goes off and reenters with PAM and BRIAN.)

LOVE AMONG THE ARTISTS

PAM: I hope it's not too late.

GERTIE: Nonsense. We're usually up to all hours.

KEITH: Are you two appearing in the final show?

PAM: They're doing a musical.

BRIAN: Kiss Me, Kate.

PAM: And neither of us sing or dance.

BRIAN: So we're just sort of filling in.

KEITH: What are your plans after it closes?

PAM: We'll be heading back to New York, I suppose.

KEITH: Are you two...?

BRIAN: A pair? Oh, no. I'm gay.

KEITH: Oh, I see.

PAM: And I've got a boy friend. He's playing the lead in Kiss Me Kate.

BRIAN: No comment.

PAM: Brian! Brian doesn't like Jeffrey, because Jeffrey gets most of the parts that Brian thinks he should be getting.

KEITH: Would you care to stay on for another week? I'll be doing Othello at the theatre, and I'm hoping to use members of the company.

LOVE AMONG THE ARTISTS

BRIAN: Well...yes.

PAM: Yes, of course.

BRIAN: What roles were you thinking of?

KEITH: I'm not quite sure. I'd like to read you both.

BRIAN: Now?

KEITH: Well, I guess now is as good a time as any. I'm afraid there's only one copy available. We'll have to share it, if you don't mind. Brian, why don't we go into my study.

BRIAN: Yes, sir.

KEITH: And if we're going to work together...

BRIAN: Yes, sir?

KEITH: Please, call me Keith. *(HE picks up the copy of Othello Gertie's been reading and starts off.)* Come along.

> *(BRIAN looks at Pam, crosses his fingers for luck, and follows KEITH off.)*

PAM: This is so exciting.

KAY: Have you ever done any Shakespeare?

PAM: I worked on some scenes. back at Northwestern. Juliet. And Rosalind in As You Like It. What part do you think I'll be reading for?

GERTIE: Desdemona, of course.

LOVE AMONG THE ARTISTS

PAM: *(To KAY)* Won't you be playing Desdemona?

KAY: No, dear. I'll be playing Emilia.

PAM: Playing with you and Keith! Of course, I don't have the role as yet.

KAY: That's true.

(KEITH reenters.)

KEITH: He's looking over the scene.

GERTIE: What are you reading him for?

KEITH: Cassio...and Iago. Though I see him really as Cassio...or Roderigo. *(To PAM)* And you'll be reading for Desdemona, of course.

GERTIE: She has worked on Shakespeare, you know. Juliet, Rosalind.

PAM: At Northwestern, and we analyzed several of the plays.

KEITH: *(HE looks at KAY.)* Are you all right?

KAY: I'm tired, dear. I'm going to turn in. Good night. *(SHE kisses KEITH, starts off, then turns to PAM.)* And good luck.

PAM: Thank you.

(KAY goes off.)

KEITH: I'm worried about her.

GERTIE: What did the doctor say?

LOVE AMONG THE ARTISTS

KEITH: He said she's doing fine, and she'll soon be up to snuff.

GERTIE: Well, there you are.

KEITH: Yes, but when?

(BRIAN appears in the doorway.)

BRIAN: I guess I'm ready.

KEITH: Okay. Let's go.

(THEY go off.)

GERTIE: Keith saw you perform, so there's nothing to worry about.

PAM: Have you ever done any Shakespeare?

GERTIE: Once. I played Celia in As You Like It, and I hated every minute of it. It's bad enough pretending to be someone else. One should, at least, be given words that people actually speak. What's this Jeffrey like?

PAM: He's bright, and very ambitious, and very good looking.

GERTIE: How long...?

PAM: Oh, we just met. This summer.

GERTIE: Ah, yes.

PAM: Was Kay, Miss Charles, in the hospital for very long?

GERTIE: She was there for a week. They took some tests and then she had a cyst removed, which turned out to be benign.

LOVE AMONG THE ARTISTS

(BRIAN reenters.)

BRIAN: *(To PAM)* It's your turn. Good luck.

PAM: Thank you. *(SHE goes off.)*

GERTIE: How did it go?

BRIAN: It's hard to tell. I never dreamt I'd be reading a scene with Keith Garrick, sitting right next to me like that. I'm hoping for Iago. Can you see me as Iago?

GERTIE: I see you as Cassio. He's a charmer.

BRIAN: I'm really a villain at heart. Of course, I can be charming...in an oily sort of way. *(After a moment)* What are you thinking?

GERTIE: I was thinking of another charmer.

BRIAN: Your husband. Did you love him very much?

GERTIE: Hmmmmm. I could have married an earl, you know, but I married Michael instead.

BRIAN: What happened to the earl?

GERTIE: I turned him over to my sister, and now my sister is a very wealthy, titled widow.

BRIAN: Was this in London?

GERTIE: Michael was an American. I came here with a revue. My sister and I were music hall performers. We sang a little and danced a little, and we were famous, in a very minor sort of way.

LOVE AMONG THE ARTISTS

I was dating Sir Henry, and then I met Michael. He was an actor, with a very promising career, and he swept me off my feet.

BRIAN: How did he die? I'm sorry.

GERTIE: That's quite all right. It was a long time ago.

BRIAN: Were you very much in love?

GERTIE: Yes, I was very much in love, and he never looked at another woman. One night Michael had a little much to drink. He left some friends at a bar, was crossing the street, and was struck down by an automobile. It took me a long time to recover, and that's when I met Kay. She and Keith were beginning to make a name for themselves. She needed a dresser, and I no longer sang or danced, and when the children came, Tony and Emily, I'd help out with the children, and gradually I became part of the family.

BRIAN: You never remarried?

GERTIE: No, dear. Like the swan, I think one falls in love, really in love, only once.

BRIAN: It's a terrible burden, isn't it?

GERTIE: What, dear? Love?

BRIAN: No, sex.

GERTIE: I sometimes think that memory is the best part of it all. There is an advantage in getting old, you know.

BRIAN: And what might that be?

GERTIE: Maybe it's because there's not that much more time left, but the world seems so much more beautiful; and the human animal, all shapes, all sizes...I gaze at them in wonder, such fascinating creatures. And it's amazing. People are so considerate with the elderly. It seems to bring out the best in them.

(PAM enters, followed by KEITH.)

KEITH: Well, that wasn't so bad, was it?

PAM: That's for you to decide. *(To BRIAN)* We should be going. We have a matinee tomorrow.

KEITH: I'm hoping to complete the casting by Monday or Tuesday.

PAM: Thank you, Mr. Garrick.

KEITH: Keith.

PAM: Keith.

BRIAN: Thank you...Keith.

PAM: Good night, Gertie. *(SHE kisses her.)*

GERTIE: Good night, dear.

BRIAN: Good night. *(HE kisses her.)*

(PAM and BRIAN go off.)

GERTIE: Well?

KEITH: Lay off.

GERTIE: You're not going to tell me.

KEITH: When I've decided, you'll be the first one to know.

LOVE AMONG THE ARTISTS

(KAY, in nightgown and robe, reenters.)

GERTIE: You're a stuffed shirt! That's what you are. *(SHE goes off.)*

KAY: Is she angry?

KEITH: She's an interfering old busybody.

KAY: You love her madly, and you know it.

KEITH: You're the one I'm in love with.

> *(HE puts his arms around her. SHE slips away and sits on the sofa. HE sits beside her and takes her hands in his.)*

KEITH: Are you up to some hanky-panky?

KAY: Not for at least a couple of weeks, I've been told. I'm sorry, dear. I feel awful.

KEITH: You mustn't feel awful. You must feel good.

KAY: I do. But I've been told to wait. *(SHE squeezes his hands and kisses him on the cheek.)*

KEITH: I think I'll go upstairs and take a nice cold shower.

> *(HE kisses her and goes off. SHE heaves a sigh, picks up the copy of OTHELLO, starts to look at it, then closes the book and tosses it away.)*

KAY: Damn! Damn, damn, damn, damn, damn!

> *(SHE sits looking forlorn as the lights come down.)*

Scene Three

(Late morning. One week later. GERTIE enters, followed by KAY then KEITH.)

KAY: I don't want to hear another word.

GERTIE: I wasn't going to say a thing.

KEITH: Why don't you calm down?

KAY: I resent your attitude. The both of you. And, for your information, I was not the one that chose that camp. And if Tony broke his leg, that might have happened anywhere.

GERTIE: I still don't understand how he broke it.

KAY: Climbing a tree, I told you. That's how he broke it! He got his foot caught somehow, and he kept twisting his leg until it fractured.

KEITH: All right, all right. Good lord! If anyone has a right to complain it's me. I'm in the middle of directing a production of Othello, and I'm the one who has to keep running back and forth.

KAY: Well, you were the one who decided to direct the production.

KEITH: I chose to direct the production because there was no one on hand that I could trust.

KAY: Then stop complaining.

KEITH: I'm not complaining. I said I have a right to complain.

KAY: About the responsibility of being a parent?

KEITH: About being married to a shrew.

LOVE AMONG THE ARTISTS

KAY: Who got excellent reviews, if you will recall.

KEITH: I'm not referring to your performance on stage.

KAY: What are you referring to? Go on! Go on! Say it!

GERTIE: Oh, stop it, you two.

KEITH: No one's accusing you of anything. Gertie, have I said anything accusatory?

KAY: Why do you keep bringing Gertie into this?

GERTIE: I'm going to start on lunch.

KAY: And for heaven's sake, please, not that damned tuna salad again.

GERTIE: *(To KEITH)* I really think the woman's gone out of her mind. *(SHE stalks off to the kitchen.)*

KEITH: You've really hurt her feelings. What is this all about?

KAY: Everything is closing in on me. And I hate the role of Emilia.

KEITH: Do you want me to replace you?

KAY: At this late date? Oh, I'll play the damn part, and I'll be brilliant.

KEITH: What are you so upset about?

KAY: I feel so useless. My children are gone. I'm not a mother anymore, and...I'm not even a woman.

LOVE AMONG THE ARTISTS

KEITH: Have you spoken to Doctor Shapiro?

KAY: How can I talk to Dr. Shapiro? He's off in the Bahamas somewhere. And you've been so patient.

KEITH: The anticipation is sometimes better than the event itself. No, no, no. I was not implying anything.

> (THEY settle on the sofa. SHE nestles her head in the crook of his arm.)

KAY: I wish you wouldn't be so nice.

KEITH: ShallI play the brute? Shall I order you about?

KAY: You did it so well as Petruchio.

KEITH: I did, didn't I?

KAY: I have nothing to hold on to.

KEITH: (HE puts his arm around her.) Hold on to me.

KAY: I remember when I first met you. He's much too nice, I thought. Completely without talent.

KEITH: And then you found out, that I wasn't really that nice, and I was loaded with talent. (HE sighs.)

KAY: How is Brian working out as Iago?

KEITH: He seems to understand the role, and he plays it intelligently, and he seems to relate to all the other actors, but there's this wall between us. It's as if he's afraid to look at me.

KAY: Have you spoken to him about it?

KEITH: I'm waiting till he's more secure with his lines. Which reminds me. I'd better look over the script. I'm expecting Pam and Brian at one. They've started to work on the set, so we can't get the stage anymore. Call me when lunch is ready.

(KEITH kisses her, and starts off. The telephone rings. KAY picks it up.)

KAY: Hello? Yes. Yes, he's here. *(To KEITH)* It's London.

(KAY hands the phone to KEITH. GERTIE appears in the doorway.)

KEITH: Hello? Hello? Roger, how are you? You got my message. Yes, we'll be playing it for a week. I hope you can you make it. Oh, good. *(HE nods and smiles at KAY.)* It'll be pretty rough, of course. Give me a ring as soon as you land. I most certainly will. Look forward. *(HE hangs up.)*

GERTIE: Was that Roger Hornsby?

KEITH: Did you know him?

GERTIE: I knew his father. A letch if there ever was one. Is he coming over?

KEITH: Yes. He's going to catch a performance, and fly right back afterwards.

GERTIE: You're still going to play him without any make up?

KEITH: That was the idea, wasn't it? *(To KAY)* He sends you his love. *(HE goes off.)*

KAY: I'm sorry if I've offended you.

LOVE AMONG THE ARTISTS

GERTIE: Don't give it a thought. You know, people are so thoughtless. No, not you. That sister of mine. I took all the trouble to send her that sweater, you'd think she would have acknowledged it somehow, a phone call, a note or...something.

KAY: Well, it's only been a week.

GERTIE: How long does it take to pick up a phone?

KAY: Why don't you call her? Maybe she's ill.

GERTIE: Lily's as healthy as a horse.

KAY: Still.

GERTIE: What time is it? *(SHE looks at her watch.)* It's too late now. I'll call her in the morning.

(KAY sits with a sigh.)

GERTIE: It hasn't been easy, I know. But it's been especially difficult for Keith, you know. And he's been so good with the children while you were away. And now the play. I don't know how he does it. I really don't, and I really don't like to interfere, but he's under tremendous pressure, and you're really not making things any easier, you know. *(Patronizing)* You really must try to be more understanding, my dear, That's a good girl.

(GERTIE pats Kay's hand condescendingly, and goes off.)

KAY: *(SHE rises, infuriated, and paces about.)* Damned bitch! *(SHE looks about, sights a figurine, picks it up and flings it to the floor, smashing it to bits.)*

(GERTIE reenters.)

79

GERTIE: What in the world was that? *(SHE sees the smashed figurine on the floor.)* Oh, my god! Ellen Terry! That was Ellen Terry. Oh, my God! What happened? Kay?

KAY: I...

GERTIE: You did that deliberately. How could you? Michael gave that to me on our tenth anniversary.

KAY: I'm sorry.

> *(GERTIE bends down and examines the pieces.)*

KAY: I'll buy you another.

GERTIE: There is no other. That was Ellen Terry as Portia. It was one of a kind.

> *(SHE rises, in tears, and walks off.)*

KAY: Gertie... I'm sorry.

> *(KAY starts to follow GERTIE when the doorbell rings. SHE goes off to answer the door. PAM and BRIAN enter, followed by KAY.)*

KAY: You're early. Have a seat. *(SHE goes off in pursuit of Gertie.)*

PAM: We're not that early.

> *(THEY sit down. The telephone rings.)*

PAM: *(After a few moments)* Do you think we ought to answer it? *(After a moment)* I'm going to answer it. *(SHE waits a few seconds then pick up the phone.)* Hello? Yes. Who? Just a moment.

LOVE AMONG THE ARTISTS

(KAY enters.)

PAM: It's for Gertie. *(SHE hands the phone to KAY.)*

KAY: Hello? Can I help you? Is it in regard to her sister? Hold on. *(SHE puts down the phone and goes to the doorway.)* Gertie. There's a phone call for you. It's from London.

PAM: Is there something wrong?

KAY: I don't know. They refuse to give me any information.

(GERTIE enters and picks up the phone.)

GERTIE: Hello? Yes, this is she. Is she...?

(GERTIE sways and almost drops the phone. KAY rushes to her side.)

GERTIE: *(SHE sits. After a moment)* When's the funeral? I'll book a flight today, or early tomorrow morning. Thank you. *(SHE hangs up and sits, in a daze.)* Pneumonia. Just like that. Maybe she never even saw the sweater. Poor Lily. Of course, she wasn't really poor. *(SHE weeps.)* I just can't believe she's gone.

(KEITH enters.)

KEITH: Did I hear the phone?

KAY: It was London. Lily's dead.

KEITH: I'm so sorry. How did it happen?

KAY: Pneumonia.

KEITH: You'll want to go over for the funeral.

81

GERTIE: Do you think I might be able to book a flight for this evening?

KEITH: We can try.

KAY: I'll help you pack.

KEITH: Why don't the two of you go out on the terrace and run lines.

BRIAN: I'm so sorry, Gertie.

GERTIE: Thank you, dear.

PAM: Is there anything we can do?

KEITH: No, no, no. We'll take care of it.

BRIAN: We'll be out on the terrace.

(PAM and BRIAN go off.)

KEITH: *(HE notices the pieces of the figurine on the floor.)* What happened here? Good Lord! Isn't that Ellen Terry?

GERTIE: As Portia.

KAY: It was an accident.

(KAY places her arm around GERTIE and leads her off. KEITH sits and picks up the phone. HE sighs and dials information.)

KEITH: *(On the phone.)* Hello? Can you give me the number for British Airlines? *(HE sighs.)* What next?

LOVE AMONG THE ARTISTS

(The lights come down as KEITH sighs and shakes his head in disbelief.)

ACT TWO

Scene One

(Late afternoon. One week later. PAM and KEITH are discovered seated. THEY have just finished rehearsing.)

KEITH: I'm not concerned about your performance. I'm concerned about you.

PAM: I'll be all right. Brian warned me, and I should have listened to him.

KEITH: I gather you and Jeffrey were having an affair.

PAM: If you can call it that. He used me, and then he tossed me aside.

KEITH: Were you in love with him?

PAM: Oh, I don't know... And, I guess I'm really to blame. What I mean to say is...he never made any promises. But he never told me that he was married. Oh, I'll get over it. I'm just angry at myself for being such a fool. And he never even bothered to say good-bye.

(KAY enters from the outside.)

KEITH: Where have you been? I was beginning to get worried.

KAY: I was at the camp. The Bemelmans were going there to visit Alfred, and they took me along. I wanted to check on Tony.

KEITH: How is he doing?

KAY: He's doing fine. His leg is in a cast. He gets around with crutches, and he's a busy as a bee.

LOVE AMONG THE ARTISTS

KEITH: There was a call for you, from Doctor Shapiro.

KAY: What did he say?

KEITH: He didn't say anything. He was just returning your call.

KAY: Did he leave a number?

KEITH: Don't you have his number?

KAY: I do not have his number in the Bahamas.

KEITH: Then call his office.

KAY: Excuse me. *(SHE goes to the phone, picks it up and dials.)* Hello? Doctor Shapiro? When did you get into town? How long will you be there? Look, Doctor, I have got to see you. I can be there in an hour. Yes, it is that important. I'll see you then. *(SHE hangs up.)* I'll call a cab.

PAM: I can drive you, if you like.

KAY: Oh, would you, dear?

KEITH: We've got a dress rehearsal tonight.

KAY: At eight o'clock. We should be back by six...six thirty.

KEITH: If you're going to go, then go.

> *(KAY kisses KEITH on the cheek and starts off as the doorbell rings.)*

KAY: I'll get it.

LOVE AMONG THE ARTISTS

(KAY goes off, followed by PAM. BRIAN enters a moment later.)

BRIAN: Where is everyone off to?

KEITH: They're going into town.

KEITH: So... How are you doing?

BRIAN: I guess that's for you to say.

KEITH: Quite, quite. How about a drink before we start?

BRIAN: A drink?

KEITH: A glass of wine. A liqueur. I have just the thing. *(HE pours two drinks, and hands one to BRIAN.)* Try this.

BRIAN: *(HE tastes the drink.)* That is good. What's it called?

KEITH: Baileys Irish Cream. I discovered it in London. of all places.

BRIAN: Have you been there often?

KEITH: Not really. We were invited to bring our production of Taming Of The Shrew to the Old Vic. And that's how this production came about. Roger Hornsby came to see our production and invited me to do Hamlet.

BRIAN: And now you're doing Othello.

KEITH: Yes, now I'm doing Othello.

BRIAN: As a Caucasian.

LOVE AMONG THE ARTISTS

KEITH: Art and politics. They really should stay out of each others way. Well, shall we?

BRIAN: Yes, sir. *(HE corrects himself.)* Keith. We decided to work on Act Three, Scene Three, the scene between Othello and Iago. You wanted to give me some notes.

KEITH: Let's just start the scene and see how it goes. Iago says, "My noble lord."

(THEY rise and position themselves.)

BRIAN: "My noble lord..."

KEITH: "What dost thou say, Iago?"

BRIAN: "Did Michael Cassio, when you woo'd my lady,
    Know of your love?"

KEITH: "He did, from first to last; why dost thou ask?"

BRIAN: "But for a satisfaction of my thoughts;
    No further harm."

KEITH: "Why of thy thoughts, Iago?

BRIAN: "I did not think he had been acquainted with her."

KEITH: "Oh, yes; and went between us very oft."

BRIAN: "Indeed!"

KEITH: "Indeed! Ay, indeed; discern'st thou ought in that?
    Is he not honest?"

BRIAN: "Honest, my lord?"

LOVE AMONG THE ARTISTS

KEITH: "Honest! Ay honest."

BRIAN: "My lord, for...."

KEITH: Let's stop there. Do you realize that all through that scene, you never looked at me once? Is there any reason why Iago would never ever look at Othello?

BRIAN: The fact of the matter is, I really don't know how to play the relationship. Iago doesn't really believe that Othello slept with his wife, nor would he be that vicious about being passed over for a promotion.

KEITH: I see. Have you had any other thoughts?

BRIAN: I think there's a love-hate relationship. As a matter of fact, I read that when Laurence Olivier played Othello with Ralph Richardson that's the way he played it.

KEITH: How?

BRIAN: As if Iago was in love with Othello.

KEITH: Oh? Well, let's try it. See where it goes. Why don't we just pick it up.
   What dost thou think?"

BRIAN: "Think, my lord?"

KEITH: "Think, my lord!
   By heaven he echoes me.
   As if there were some monster in his thought
   Too hideous to be shown. Thou dost mean something.
   I heard thee say, even now, thou likedst not that
   When Cassio left my wife; what did'st not like?
   And when I told thee he was of my counsel

LOVE AMONG THE ARTISTS

In my whole course of wooing, though criedst, 'Indeed!
And didst contract and purse thy brow together,
As if thou then hadst shut up in thy brain
Some horrible conceit; if thou dost love me,
Show me thy thought."

BRIAN: *(Who's been eyeing him with love, places his hand on KEITH's cheek, moves close and kisses him.)* "My lord, you know I love you." *(HE kisses KEITH again, passionately.)*

KEITH: Brian...? I...

(KEITH stands, perplexed and disturbed, disturbed by his growing response. BRIAN runs his hand along Keith's arms, his shoulders, his thigh and kisses him again as the lights come down.)

Scene Two

(Early afternoon, the following day. KAY enters with GERTIE from the interior.)

GERTIE: It's good to be back.

KAY: We missed you.

GERTIE: How is Keith doing?

KAY: I still think it was a mistake for him to star and direct.

GERTIE: I'm sure he'll be fine. And how are my two young proteges coming along?

KAY: Pam is quite lovely.

GERTIE: And Brian?

KAY: Keith was a bit concerned about him, but he seem's to be coming along.

GERTIE: And the children?

KAY: Emily won a silver cup for archery, and Tony's still, hobbling around on crutches, but he seems to be enjoying himself. And yesterday I finally cornered Doctor Shapiro.

GERTIE: And?

KAY: I'm fit as a fiddle, and ready for love. You haven't said a thing. How did it go?

GERTIE: I think it's time for my Scotch. What can I get you?

KAY: Nothing. Tonight **is** the opening.

LOVE AMONG THE ARTISTS

GERTIE: *(SHE pours herself a drink.)* I've decided I'm not going to be buried. I will not be placed in a coffin, lowered into a deep hole in the ground, and have people shoveling dirt on top of me. In addition to that, it was drizzling. There were some bright spots though. Several friends from the dear, dead past came out of the woodwork. There was Henry Ainley. He was a handsome leading man, the last time I laid eyes on him. "Henry, dear," I said, "what happened to your hair?" "It's in a box," he said. "And, unfortunately, I forgot to take it out this morning." And poor dear Lily. Laying there in that elegant coffin, dressed to the nines. It's sinful the way they make up corpses. But then again, why not? It's all make-believe, is it not? Who would have thought that I'd end up here, in the wilds of Massachusetts, as a widowed refugee from the English Music Hall?

KAY: You're not a refugee. You're a member, a beloved member, of a loving family. Drink your Scotch, and stop feeling sorry for yourself.

> *(GERTIE sighs, and takes a sip of her Scotch as KEITH enters from the outside.)*

KEITH: Good Lord! She's hardly landed, and she's guzzling her Scotch.

GERTIE: You would, too, if you had to bury your sister.

KEITH: Good morning, Love. *(HE kisses her.)* And welcome home.

GERTIE: Where have you been all morning?

KEITH: Technical rehearsal. I need a drink. One small one. *(HE pours himself a short Scotch and takes a sip.)*

KAY: How did the rehearsal go?

LOVE AMONG THE ARTISTS

KEITH: That young man on the lights makes me very nervous.

KAY: Have you heard from Roger Hornsby?

KEITH: He called me from Boston. He's going straight to the theatre, and catching a plane immediately after the performance. *(To GERTIE.)* I want to hear all about the funeral, but not now. I've got to take a nap. Wake me at seven. *(HE kisses KAY, then kisses GERTIE.)* Welcome home. *(HE goes off.)*

GERTIE: Has he lost weight?

KAY: I know. Thank God there's almost a month before he leaves for London. Would you like me to help you unpack?

GERTIE: No, no, no. I've brought all sorts of goodies, and I don't want you to see them...as yet. When are the children due home?

(The telephone rings. KAY picks up the phone.)

KAY: Hello? *(To GERTIE)* It's them. *(Back on the phone)* Tony? Is anything wrong? Oh, how sweet of you! Thank you for thinking of us. Daddy's taking a nap right now. Of course, I'll tell him. Thank you, Emily. Daddy's sleeping, but I'll tell him you called. There's someone here who wants to say hello. *(To GERTIE)* I'm going to start on dinner. *(SHE hand the phone to GERTIE and goes off.)*

GERTIE: Hello, Sweetie. It was all very sad, and I'm glad to be back. Well, of course I'm going to the opening. Now, what have you two been up to while I've been gone? I want to hear all about it.

(The lights come down as GERTIE listens on the phone.)

Scene Three

(Mid-morning. One week later. The doorbell rings. The doorbell rings again. KAY, wearing a housecoat enters from the interior, goes off to answer the door and reenters with PAM.)

KAY: You're up bright and early.

PAM: Did I wake you?

KAY: Not really, no. I'm still asleep. What time is it?

PAM: Ten o'clock.

KAY: There ought to be a law against closing night parties. What's happening?

PAM: I'm off to Paris.

KAY: Paris?! Goodness me.

PAM: I've got a part in a movie. When I got home last night, there was a call from Mr. Hornsby in London. They're three hours ahead of us, you know. And they're shooting this movie about the Americans in Paris in the nineteen twenties, and they want me to play Zelda, Zelda Fitzgerald. She's got two scenes.

KAY: Have you ever done any film work?

PAM: I did some extra work to help pay the rent, and I did a walk on once with two lines. But this is a real part, in a major movie.

KAY: I think it's wonderful. Incidentally, when Mr. Hornsby called, did he say anything at about the production?

PAM: Why no. Why do you ask?

93

LOVE AMONG THE ARTISTS

KAY: Well, he left so suddenly.

PAM: Well, he did have a plane to catch. Is Keith awake, by any chance?

KAY: What's that? Yes, of course. We're busy packing. I'll fetch him.

> *(KAY goes off. PAM walks about the room, remembering her first visit, the antique she touched, the ash tray in which she placed the cigar. KEITH enters.)*

KEITH: Good morning.

PAM: Good morning. I'm off to Paris.

KEITH: So I've been told. Congratulations.

PAM: Thank you.

KEITH: When Mr. Hornsby called you, Did he say anything at all about the production?

PAM: No. But I'm sure he was pleased.

KEITH: Yes. Yes, of course, and I think you'll make a lovely Zelda.

PAM: It's my first real part in a movie. It's not the thee-a-tah, of course. *(With exaggerated elegance.)* But even if I become a movie star, I shall always return to the "thee-a-tah". And I want to thank you, for giving me the privilege of working with you and Kay. It's been the most exciting thing that has ever happened to me in my whole life.

LOVE AMONG THE ARTISTS

KEITH: And I'm sure there are many more exciting things to come.

(SHE hugs and kisses him as KAY enters.)

KAY: Here, here, here! What's going on?

(PAM rushes to KAY and hugs and kisses her.)

PAM: It's all so wonderful.

KAY: You will keep in touch.

PAM: I'll send you all the details. The good, the bad and the ugly. I just can't believe this is happening to me. Working with the two of you. Doing a movie in Paris. It's like a dream come true.

KAY: Hold onto that dream, my dear, if you can.

(GERTIE enters from the terrace, removing a working glove and carrying a pair of shears.)

GERTIE: What's going on?

PAM: I'm going to be in a movie in Paris.

GERTIE: Well, of course you are.

PAM: Mr. Hornsby. He called me last night, all the way from London. I'll be playing Zelda Fitzgerald in this movie about the Americans in Paris in the nineteen twenties, and I've got two scenes. *(PAM rushes over to GERTIE, hugs and kisses her.)*

GERTIE: Goodness me!

PAM: Isn't it exciting?!

LOVE AMONG THE ARTISTS

GERTIE: And you're going to write us all about it.

PAM: Oh, I will, I will. I better be going. I've still got to finish packing. I've got to get to Boston by five. That's when my plane leaves for Paris. Can you believe it? Wish me luck.

GERTIE, KEITH & KAY: Good luck!

(PAM throws them a kiss as rushes off.)

KEITH: *(After a moment)* Not a word! Not one single word!

GERTIE: About what?

KEITH: About what! About my performance, for God's sake, about my playing Othello in white face. Oh, never mind! *(HE stalks off.)*

KAY: I don't understand it. I really don't.

GERTIE: I told you, my dear. He enjoyed the show, and he said he would be in touch. Kay, for heaven's sake. The man is an artistic director of a major theatrical company. In addition to that, he's shooting a movie.

KAY: I'm aware of that. The fact of the matter is, this whole production, this whole thing was arranged for his benefit.

GERTIE: Will you relax! He will call you eventually. He has to give you a rehearsal date.

KAY: You're right. You're absolutely right. *(SHE heaves a sigh. After a moment)* I'm so happy for Pamela. Do you remember being that young? Which reminds me. Stay right where you are. *(SHE runs off and returns with a package.)* This is for you. Open it.

LOVE AMONG THE ARTISTS

GERTIE: *(SHE opens the package and removes the gift.)* It's a pen and inkwell set.

KAY: It belonged to Ellen Terry. You hate it. And I went to all that trouble. I searched out every shop in Boston. It's very rare, you know, and, I might add, very expensive. You don't care for it.

GERTIE: It's...very interesting.

KAY: Oh, damn!

GERTIE: *(SHE embraces Kay and kisses her.)* It was very sweet of you. And I shall cherish it; not because it belonged to Ellen Terry, but because it came from you...with love. Thank you. I'm going to take it right to my room, and place it in a very special spot.

(GERTIE starts off as the doorbell rings.)

KAY: I'll get it.

(GERTIE goes off. KAY goes off and returns with BRIAN.)

BRIAN: I've come to say good-bye.

KAY: Where are you off to?

BRIAN: The big city. New York, that is. That's where I'm from, at the moment. I want to thank you, to thank you both for the privilege of working with you.

KAY: You were very good. Brian. And I'm sure you're going to have a great future. I think Keith would like a word with you. Don't go 'way.

LOVE AMONG THE ARTISTS

(KAY goes off. BRIAN paces about, sits, looks about the room, sighs and remains lost in thought. GERTIE reenters.)

GERTIE: So, there you are. My favorite Thespian.

BRIAN: I've come to say good-bye.

GERTIE: Where are you off to?

BRIAN: Back to New York, to make the rounds, to face the future.

GERTIE: How would you like to come to London with me? I'm very wealthy now, you know, and I'll need a secretary, or some sort of assistant, to help me manage the estate. It worked out perfectly, my dear. I turned Sir Henry down, and now I'm inheriting all his money, and I didn't even have to put up with him.

BRIAN: Would you really like me to come with you? What I mean to say is, it would be a golden opportunity. Before he left, Mr. Hornsby sent me a note backstage. If I ever come to London, he wrote, be sure to look him up. He didn't offer me a job, of course, but apparently, he did think highly enough of my performance to send me that note.

GERTIE: If he bothered to send you a note, then I'm sure he would be of use.

(KEITH enters.)

GERTIE: Brian is coming to London with me.

BRIAN: Actually, Mr. Hornsby sent me a note backstage. And I thought I might try my luck in London.

GERTIE: Which reminds me, I must get a letter off to the lawyer.

98

LOVE AMONG THE ARTISTS

(To BRIAN) I'm taking you to lunch at the Inn. Meet me there at one.

BRIAN: Okay.

    (GERTIE goes off.)

KEITH: By the way, what did Mr. Hornsby say?

BRIAN: What's that?

KEITH: In that note he sent you?

BRIAN: Nothing much, really. He enjoyed my performance, and if I was ever in London, to be sure to look him up

KEITH: I see. Incidentally...

BRIAN: Yes, sir?

KEITH: Really, Brian.

BRIAN: It's just that...

KEITH: What?

BRIAN: I don't know what our relationship is exactly.

KEITH: The fact of the matter is, I've been meaning to have a talk with you, Brian. That afternoon.... The fact of the matter is... I was irresponsible...and, as a matter of fact, rather horny. Kay has had some health problems, you see...and was not available for...too long a time.

BRIAN: I see...

KEITH: I'm sorry if I may have misled you. It should never have happened, and I owe you an apology. You were going to say...?

BRIAN: I was just wondering...

KEITH: Yes? Go on.

BRIAN: If you're not fooling yourself.

KEITH: You think, perhaps, I'm gay.

BRIAN: You're the one who brought it up.

KEITH: The fact of the matter is, I tried it once, very briefly, a long time ago.

BRIAN: And?

KEITH: It's not for me.

BRIAN: I see. But that afternoon...

KEITH: "Any port in a storm," dear boy. I'm sorry if you thought it was anything more. I'm really very fond of you, Brian. and you're a fine actor.

BRIAN: Thank you.

KEITH: And...

BRIAN: What?

KEITH: I hate to sound corny...but...can we be...friends...? *(HE extends his hand.)*

BRIAN: Man to man?

LOVE AMONG THE ARTISTS

KEITH: Man To Man.

(THEY shake hands.)

KEITH: And I think, that when you get to London, good things will come your way.

BRIAN: Thank you, Keith. *(HE embraces him.)* That was just a friendly hug. And maybe we'll be running into each other in London.

KEITH: I'm sure we will.

(BRIAN goes off. KEITH sighs and sits lost in thought. KAY enters.)

KAY: How did it go?

KEITH: What's that? Needless to say, it was not my finest hour. But no, you were right. It was the right thing to do. Tell me something...

KAY: Yes?

KEITH: Have you ever had sex with a woman?

KAY: Not really, no. I have had a crush or two. I wouldn't worry about it, dear.

KEITH: What I am really worried about is the fact that I haven't heard a word from Roger. He sends a note backstage to Brian, telling him how much he enjoyed his performance. He puts in a call to Pam in the middle of the night, to hire her for a film to shoot in Paris. The fact of the matter is, he came all the way over here to see my performance as Othello, and he hasn't said a word, not one single word.

LOVE AMONG THE ARTISTS

KAY: Do you really like Othello, dear? I mean I'm so sick of blood and gore. That's all one reads about, that's all one hears. I like plays about life...what does Chekhov say?...about life, life as it ought to be?

(The phone rings.)

KAY: I'll get it. *(SHE picks up the phone.)* Hello? Roger, it's so nice to hear from you. Hold on. It's the master himself.

KEITH: And about time, too. *(HE takes the phone.)* Hello, Roger. Oh, I know how busy you are. Thank you. And by the way, what did you think of my take on Othello? I mean not blacking up? Ah, yes. So you said. We must keep up with the times. Incidentally, are you planning to tinker with any of the lines? Well, it does refer to Othello as black. Yes, of course. October first. Right. I most certainly will. *(HE hangs up.)* Can you believe it? He's cutting all the lines, *(After a moment)* What do you think?

KAY: About what?

KEITH: About what!! You know perfectly well about what?

KAY: There were no complaints from the audience about a white Othello.

KEITH: Yes, well, there was one English teacher. I forget his name. He thought that maybe I ran out of makeup. My first appearance in London in a Royal Shakespeare production....or...

KAY: Or what?

KEITH: My integrity, that's what. Kay, he wants to cut the heart of the play. It's so...phoney, so...meretricious.

KAY: Meretricious?

LOVE AMONG THE ARTISTS

KEITH: Lack of integrity, that's what it is. Bowing to the fashion of the times. What do you think I ought to do?

KAY: Don't look at me.

KEITH: I'm asking you, What do you think I ought to do?

KAY: Keith, you have always made up your mind, no matter what I say.

KEITH: I'm asking you.

KAY: I think you ought to...

KEITH: Yes?

KAY: Do what you think you ought to do.

KEITH: Thanks a lot.

> (*KEITH sighs, and stands thinking, as the lights come down.*)

THE ROAD NOT TAKEN
A Bi-Sexual Comedy

CAST OF CHARACTERS

Jeff Carter

Audrey Wingate

Don Carter

Eve Beardsly

SCENE
New York City: Jeff Carter's apartment in The Village.

TIME
Early Autumn
1980

Two roads diverged in a yellow wood,
And sorry, I could not travel both
Robert Frost, "The Road Not Taken"

ACT ONE

Scene One

(Early evening. The living room of Jeff Carter's apartment in The Village. It's a sparsely furnished room. Some pictures cut out from newspapers, or magazines, are tacked on a wall; pictures of Dostoevski, Tolstoy, Ernest Hemingway and Thomas Wolfe. The doorbell rings. It rings twice. AUDREY WINGATE, an attractive woman on her early thirties, enters from the interior. SHE stands hesitantly. The doorbell rings for the third time. SHE opens the door. DON CARTER, a pleasant looking man in his early thirties, is discovered. HE's holding a large suitcase.)

AUDREY: Can I help you? *(Studies him)*You're Don, aren't you?

DON: And you must be...

AUDREY: Audrey.

DON: Yes, Audrey. Jeff never told me how attractive you were.

AUDREY: Thank you.

DON: May I come in?

AUDREY: I'm sorry. *(SHE steps aside.)*

DON: This suitcase is kind of heavy.

AUDREY: What have you got in there?

DON: My worldly goods.

AUDREY: Are you moving?

THE ROAD NOT TAKEN

DON: I'm always on the move. I'm an itinerant player, you know.

AUDREY: Yes, of course. I know all about you.

DON: I certainly hope not.

AUDREY: You're back from....

DON: Five weeks in Idaho.

AUDREY: Was it successful?

DON: That's a good question. Was it worthwhile? Definitely. Did I make any money? Enough to live on. I gather my little brother isn't in at the moment.

AUDREY: No. No, he isn't.

DON: Do you know when he'll be back?

AUDREY: Actually he's been taking this literature class at NYU, and he doesn't get back till about eight or nine.

DON: I gather he said nothing to you about his putting me up here for a while.

AUDREY: No. No, he hasn't. Actually I have a confession to make. I really shouldn't be here.

DON: Oh?

AUDREY: No. Well, you see, Jeff and I have sort of split up.

DON: I'm sorry to hear that. He spoke so highly of you. I'm terribly thirsty. What is there to drink?

THE ROAD NOT TAKEN

AUDREY: There's some wine. I think....or some ginger ale.

DON: Ginger ale would be fine.

AUDREY: I'll take a look.

> *(AUDREY goes off. DON takes in the apartment. AUDREY returns with a can of ginger ale and a glass.)*

DON: Thank you.

AUDREY: Where do you go from here?

DON: For the moment, I don't go anywhere. The first thing I've got to do is pick up a copy of Backstage, and see where my future lies. What do you do, may I ask?

AUDREY: I'm a librarian.

DON: You're much too attractive for a librarian.

AUDREY: Thank you.

DON: You think you and Jeff might possibly get together again?

AUDREY: Not unless some major changes take place.

DON: Like what?

AUDREY: I believe in facing facts. I can't go through life closing my eyes and pretending.

DON: And you think Jeff can?

AUDREY: I think he's fooling himself; pretending to be a writer; pretending to be a novelist. He hangs out with the so-called intelligentsia, leading this so-called Bohemian life, which consists of a lot of talk, most of it phoney, and a huge amount of drinking. Meanwhile I don't think he's written a single word. He insists that he has, but when I ask to see it, he says it's not ready yet. And besides, he says, I'm too critical.

DON: Maybe he's not ready to show it to anyone.

AUDREY: He's been at it for over two years. You've heard of Carlton Advertising.

DON: Yes, of course. As a matter of fact I auditioned for them once, for a commercial.

AUDREY: Well, the vice president is a cousin of mine, and I took the trouble to make a copy of this paper Jeff wrote on Thomas Wolfe.

DON: Yes, I've read it.

AUDREY: Well, I gave it to my cousin, and he was so impressed with it that he offered Jeff a job as copy writer.

DON: And Jeff turned it down.

AUDREY: I think he's just fooling himself.

DON: By the way, you don't happen to know of any apartments that might be available. I'm welcome here, I know, but brotherly love can go so far, and this place is kind of small.

AUDREY: Actually I'm planning to move out of mine in about a week or so.

DON: Oh?

THE ROAD NOT TAKEN

AUDREY: I live upstairs, you know.

DON: Yes, I know.

AUDREY: And my apartment's almost as small as this one, and there's a larger one opening up on my floor.

DON: Can I take a look at it?

AUDREY: Right now?

DON: If that's all right with you.

AUDREY: Sure. Why not?

DON: What'll I do with my bag?

AUDREY: Why don't you leave it in the so-called bedroom.

DON: Okay. *(HE goes off with the suitcase and returns.)* When did you say you were moving out?

AUDREY: Some time next week. *(SHE opens the door.)* Be careful. The light's out in the hallway and it's pretty dark.

> *(DON picks up his drink and follows AUDREY off. After a few moments the door is opened. EVE BEARDSLY, a pretty girl in her early twenties, is escorted into the room by JEFF CARTER, an attractive man in his mid twenties.)*

JEFF: This is it, such as it is.

EVE: It's so dark out there.

JEFF: From the dark into the light. Come to think of it, I don't remember leaving my lights on.

THE ROAD NOT TAKEN

EVE: Have you been here long?

JEFF: What's that? Two years. Can I get you a drink?

EVE: Some white wine, perhaps?

JEFF: I don't have any white. I have a merlot.

EVE: Okay.

JEFF: *(HE indicates the sofa.)* Make yourself comfortable.

EVE: *(SHE walks about, inspecting the room.)* I really shouldn't be here.

JEFF: *(HE pours the wine.)* Why not?

EVE: I see you have a picture of Thomas Wolfe. Is he a favorite of yours?

JEFF: Have you read "Look Homeward, Angel."?

EVE: Yes, of course.

JEFF: I was blown away. I wrote a term paper once on Thomas Wolfe, and he paid me a visit. His ghost that is.

EVE: Oh?

JEFF: This was during my senior year. I was coming up the stairs at this boarding house I was staying at, and there was an open window on the landing. I felt this breeze coming though the window, and suddenly I was confronted by the ghost of Thomas Wolfe.

EVE: Did you actually see him?

JEFF: No exactly, no. But he was there. I could feel his presence, standing right there in front of me.

EVE: What did you do?

JEFF: Nothing. I was startled, at first. I was afraid he might resent my poking into his private life. But then, I had the feeling that he was there to pay me a visit. It was really weird. My hair actually stood on end.

EVE: How long did he stay?

JEFF: Just long enough to let me know that he approved. At least that was the feeling I had. *(HE hands her the wine.)*

EVE: Thank you.

JEFF: Have you ever been visited by any ghosts?

EVE: Not really. Jane Austen's my favorite. And I do like Willa Cather.

JEFF: *(HE pours a Scotch.)* One of my favorite movies is that old Pride And Prejudice with Greer Garson and Laurence Olivier.

EVE: I see you've got Dostoevski on your wall.

JEFF: Dostoevski's the reason I decided to become a writer. When I read Crime And Punishment, I was blown away. And Somerset Maugham; he really knows how to tell a story. *(HE sits on the sofa.)*

EVE: How many rooms do you have?

JEFF: Just the one, and an alcove which is my bedroom, and the walk in kitchen.

THE ROAD NOT TAKEN

EVE: Well, I guess that's enough for one person. I mean, you do live alone.

JEFF: For the moment. I keep hoping I can lure some lovely young maiden to move in with me.

EVE: Where would she stay?

JEFF: Here with me.

EVE: Yes, of course.

JEFF: We would share. We'd take turns cooking, not that there's much of a kitchen. As a matter of fact, there's only room for one person at a time.

EVE: Do you cook?

JEFF: I can roast a chicken. I can make an omelet. I can dish up a mean salad. Do you...cook?

EVE: Not very well.

JEFF: This sofa's very comfortable.

(SHE sits down on the far end of the sofa, stiff and erect.)

JEFF: You're not from Boston, are you?

EVE: Why do you ask?

JEFF: There's something rather Bostonian about you, something prim and proper.

EVE: Oh, dear. Is that the way I come across?

THE ROAD NOT TAKEN

JEFF: Not that it isn't completely charming.

EVE: Thank you, I think. Are you enjoying the class?

JEFF: Yes. Yes, I am. Apparently the Old Testament is much more violent and erotic than the New.

EVE: Why did you sign up for it?

JEFF: Actually I'm just auditing the class. David's an old friend of mine and he invited me to sit in. And you?

EVE: I was sent here on a fellowship, and that course was one of the reasons. I'm curious....

JEFF: Yes?

EVE: All during the course, you never said one word to me. And then these last two weeks you've suddenly become...so friendly.

JEFF: Is that bad?

EVE: No, of course not. I just wonder why it took you so long.

JEFF: Well, actually, I was involved with someone.

EVE: And now you're no longer involved?

JEFF: All good things must come to an end.

EVE: Why? Why must they come to an end?

JEFF: Are you involved?

EVE: I asked you first.

THE ROAD NOT TAKEN

JEFF: I guess I realized that the two of us weren't suited for one another.

(The doorbell rings.)

EVE: That was the doorbell.

JEFF: I'm really not expecting anyone.

(The doorbell rings again.)

EVE: Aren't you going to answer it?

JEFF: I guess I'd better.

(HE goes to the door and opens it. DON is discovered.)

DON: Is this the abode of the successor to Ernest Hemingway and F. Scott Fitzgerald?

JEFF: This is the home of the original Jeff Carter.

DON: Might a poor humble player enter your abode?

JEFF: Mi casa, su casa.

DON: Are you quite sure?

JEFF: Did I get it wrong?

DON: I don't know. I never took Spanish.

JEFF: That was Spanish? I thought it was Italian. Why are you standing there? Welcome, welcome.

THE ROAD NOT TAKEN

DON: *(HE enters.)* Thank you. You have a visitor. A pretty one at that.

JEFF: *(Closing the door)* This is Eve.

DON: *(In mock astonishment)* Really?

JEFF: Enough already. *(To EVE)* As you may have gathered by now, or maybe not, this is my wandering brother. My older brother, star of stage, screen.

DON: Only stage. I'm Don.

EVE: How do you do? Are you an actor?

JEFF: A brilliant actor.

DON: You're only saying that because it's true.

JEFF: How was your summer?

DON: Interesting.

JEFF: Just interesting?

DON: I learned something.

JEFF: What did you learn?

DON: Comedy technique.

JEFF: At this late date?

DON: You're never too old to learn.

JEFF: Where's your luggage?

THE ROAD NOT TAKEN

DON: In your bedroom. Pardon me, your alcove.

JEFF: How did it get there?

DON: A former friend of yours let me in.

JEFF: She was here?

DON: She'd have to be, if she let me in.

JEFF: That's interesting.

EVE: I should be going. I'm sure you two have a great deal to talk about.

JEFF: Don and I will have plenty of time to talk.

DON: And, if you leave, I'll feel guilty. Where did you meet this brother of mine?

EVE: In this class we're both taking?

DON: *(To JEFF)* You're taking a class?

JEFF: I'm auditing.

DON: What are you auditing?

JEFF: The Old Testament.

DON: You're not serious? Didn't you get enough of the new?

EVE: Actually the Old Testament is very colorful.

JEFF: My brother's an atheist.

DON: Wrong. I'm an agnostic. Actually my philosophy is that of Noel Coward's. "I believe in being kind to everyone, and giving money to old beggar women, and being as gay as possible." Gay, that is, in the more classical sense of the word.

EVE: I'd love some coffee. Do you have coffee?

JEFF: I have coffee. I have tea. I've even got a coffee maker.

EVE: Would anyone else care for some coffee?

DON: That might be nice.

EVE: The kitchen...?

JEFF: Through there.

EVE: I'll find it. *(SHE goes off.)*

DON: Charming. Is that the replacement?

JEFF: Hopefully.

DON: So, how's the novel coming?

JEFF: What did Audrey have to say?

DON: About your novel?

JEFF: About me? About us?

DON: She thinks there is no novel. She thinks you're just fooling yourself, that you don't really want to be a writer, that you just want to enjoy being a glamorous bohemian.

JEFF: Is that what she said?

THE ROAD NOT TAKEN

DON: In so many words. *(After a moment)* Are you okay?

JEFF: Yes! Yes, I'm fine!

DON: Okay, okay.

JEFF: She really gets under my skin.

DON: Then the feelings must run deep.

JEFF: I feel sorry for her.

DON: Pity and love, they're almost the same, you know.

JEFF: Let's talk about you.

DON: Is there a novel, or isn't there?

JEFF: If you must know, there is.

DON: Good. Not good.

(JEFF sighs.)

DON: How far have you gotten?

JEFF: I have the outline in my head, and I've written part of the first chapter.

DON: That's a start. What's the problem?

JEFF: I'm stuck.

DON: Why do you think that is?

THE ROAD NOT TAKEN

JEFF: I know why it is. Because I realize that when, and if, I ever finish the book, I couldn't possibly show it to anyone.

DON: Why?

JEFF: Because it's about the family.

DON: Well, they say to write about what you know. Why couldn't you show it to anyone?

JEFF: Because it would offend a lot of people.

DON: So what?

JEFF: I just couldn't do that.

DON: Jeff, dear boy, you can't make an omelet without breaking some eggs.

JEFF: Did you just think that up?

DON: It's one of many words of wisdom I've stored over the years.

JEFF: I'd have to show what sort of a bully Aunt Edna is, what a braggart and what an egotist. I'd have to tell how cousin Frank went to jail for forgery and embezzlement, and how Uncle Rudy's continually unfaithful to Aunt Lucy, and she pretends that he's the ideal husband. Enough of my problem. What about yours?

DON: Oy, doctor, have I got problems!

JEFF: You've converted to Judaism.

DON: That would involve circumcision, and I shudder at the very thought.

THE ROAD NOT TAKEN

JEFF: Has the divorce come through?

DON: A few weeks ago.

JEFF: You said you were going to contest it.

DON: I decided not to.

JEFF: Why?

DON: I didn't see the point.

JEFF: If you love her?

DON: I guess I love the theatre more.

JEFF: You had to make a choice? Did she ask you to?

DON: As a matter of fact, the last time we met, I said I would give it up. I said I'd get a full time job, just like any normal human being; and even as I said it, we both knew it wouldn't work. Last year I took a full time job as a clerk in this government office, and I thought I'd go out of my mind. The fact of the matter is, she wants a family. She wants security. She wants children.

JEFF: Maybe you ought to give it a try.

DON: I just can't. Theatre is what I live for.

JEFF: Well, maybe you did the right thing. Maybe, in the long run, she'll be the loser.

DON: Cold comfort that would be.

(EVE reenters.)

THE ROAD NOT TAKEN

EVE: I couldn't find the coffee maker. I looked high and now.

JEFF: It's on the top shelf.

DON: I am absolutely starved. Do you have any food in the house?

JEFF: I wasn't expecting to feed you at this very moment.

DON: You see what a brother I have? He'd let his beloved sibling starve to death in front of his very eyes.

JEFF: Why don't we go out? *(To EVE)* Are you hungry?

EVE: A little.

JEFF: Is Monte's okay?

EVE: That would be fine.

JEFF: Why don't you two go on ahead? I've got a quick call to make.

DON: Be kind.

> *(DON goes off with EVE. JEFF picks up the phone and dials.)*

JEFF: Audrey, would you come down here for a minute, please. Yes, now. I'd appreciate it. Thank you.

> *(HE hangs up, paces about, takes a sip of his drink, then paces. The doorbell rings. JEFF opens the door and AUDREY enters.)*

AUDREY: What is it?

THE ROAD NOT TAKEN

JEFF: What, may I ask, were you doing in my apartment?

AUDREY: I came down to pick up some of my things.

JEFF: Like what?

AUDREY: Like some books, and records.

JEFF: I thought you didn't have any room for all those things.

AUDREY: I will have soon. I'm moving.

JEFF: Where?

AUDREY: To a larger apartment.

JEFF: You're leaving town?

AUDREY: No, I'm not leaving town.

JEFF: I just asked you a simple question.

AUDREY: And I gave you a simple answer. What do you want to know?

JEFF: All right. Keep your secrets.

AUDREY: There are no secrets. The Blackstones are moving out, and I'm taking over their apartment.

JEFF: That's a two bedroom apartment. What do you need a two bedroom apartment for?

AUDREY: I want to stretch out. Is there anything wrong with that?

JEFF: Are you going to be sharing it with anyone?

THE ROAD NOT TAKEN

AUDREY: And suppose I was? What business is it of yours?

JEFF: Oh, now look...

AUDREY: What?

JEFF: Just because we're no longer...

AUDREY: Lovers?

JEFF: I still consider you a friend.

AUDREY: How touching!

JEFF: Don't be like that.

AUDREY: Like what?

JEFF: Are you feeling all right?

AUDREY: Yes. I'm feeling fine.

JEFF: You look sort of peaked.

AUDREY: You don't look so hot yourself.

JEFF: Well, if you're gonna act like that?

AUDREY: Like what?

JEFF: If you need any help...in moving, let me know.

AUDREY: Thank you.

JEFF: I don't understand you, I really don't.

THE ROAD NOT TAKEN

AUDREY: And vice versa.

JEFF: You know, Audrey, no matter how close a relationship is, there's got to be space. There are certain areas that are private.

AUDREY: I have never tried to invade your...space. I think I've given you plenty of space. I've put up with your moods, your stubbornness, your nastiness.

JEFF: When have I ever been nasty?

AUDREY: Ha!

JEFF: When?

AUDREY: I am not a nosy bitch.

JEFF: I'm sorry, but sometimes you do get under my skin.

AUDREY: A very thin skin, I might add.

JEFF: Okay, okay. So I'm sensitive. Is that a crime?

AUDREY: Oh, look. This is pointless. If you want your key back, I will give it to you, as soon as I collect my things.

JEFF: Don't you think I should have been consulted about you taking your things? I mean some of those books and some of those records are mine, and I should like to be here when you decide to help yourself.

AUDREY: All right. Let's get started.

JEFF: I can't right now. I have someone waiting for me.

AUDREY: Anyone I know?

THE ROAD NOT TAKEN

JEFF: No.

AUDREY: I was just asking.

JEFF: My brother and a friend. And the friend is female, if that's what you want to know.

AUDREY: Good. And I hope you treat her with more respect than you did me. Is there anything else?

JEFF: Not at the moment.

AUDREY: Well, when you do find the time, please let me know.

JEFF: I will do that little thing. Stay well.

AUDREY: You, too. *(SHE starts off.)*

JEFF: What?

AUDREY: I didn't say a thing.

> *(AUDREY goes off. JEFF sighs, stands lost in thought, shakes his head, turns off the lights and goes off as the stage lights come down.)*

Scene Two

(Three hours later. The door is opened and EVE enters, followed by JEFF.)

EVE: Why is it so dark out there?

(JEFF turns on the lights.)

EVE: And so light in here?

JEFF: Because I have magic.

EVE: You're a magician.

JEFF: "Yes, I have tricks in my pocket. I have things up my sleeve." Tennessee Williams. The Glass Menagerie.

EVE: It's been a lovely evening. I like your brother.

JEFF: More than me?

EVE: He seems so sad.

JEFF: He's just been divorced.

EVE: Oh, what a pity!

JEFF: He'll get over it.

(SHE sighs.)

JEFF: Now that was a sigh. What were you thinking about?

EVE: I was thinking about Ohio.

JEFF: What about it?

THE ROAD NOT TAKEN

EVE: Because in two weeks time that's where I'll be, back in Ohio.

JEFF: Must you go back?

EVE: That's where I live.

JEFF: No!

.EVE: No? Where **do** I live?

JEFF: *(HE points to his head.)* Up here. *(HE points to his heart.)* In here.

EVE: If only that were true. If only I had the courage that you have, to pursue ones dream.

JEFF: Do you have a dream?

EVE: I did once, when I was a little girl.

JEFF: And what was your dream?

> *(SHE laughs.)*

JEFF: It must have been a funny dream.

EVE: I dreamt...

JEFF: What?

EVE: I was a princess, a lovely princess in a beautiful white dress, with a tiara on my long, long hair.

JEFF: And Prince Charming came and swept you off your feet.

EVE: You had the same dream?

THE ROAD NOT TAKEN

JEFF: No. I dreamt...

EVE: What did you dream?

JEFF: I dreamt I was a frog.

EVE: A frog?

JEFF: A frog, and a beautiful princess in a beautiful white gown, with long flowing hair bent over and...

EVE: And what?

JEFF: And kissed me.

EVE: And...?

JEFF: I turned into a handsome prince.

> *(JEFF leans forward, prepared to kisses her. SHE pulls away.)*

EVE: I really shouldn't be here.

JEFF: Why:

EVE: Because I'm sort of engaged.

JEFF: Sort of?

EVE: Sort of.

JEFF: No ring?

EVE: No ring.

THE ROAD NOT TAKEN

JEFF: Who is this rival of mine?

EVE: He's a professor. He claims to be one, at any rate. In actuality he's only an associate professor, newly appointed at that.

JEFF: A mere child.

EVE: Oh God, no! He's old. He's an old, old man.

JEFF: How old is he?

EVE: In years, you mean? In years he's thirty. In actuality, he's, at least, fifty or maybe even sixty.

JEFF: That is old.

EVE: That's what I said. He's an old, old man. Would you want to be married to an old, old man?

JEFF: That thought never crossed my mind.

EVE: Well, think about it. That's what I've been doing, thinking about it, and thinking about it, and thinking about it. Do I really want to be married to that old, old man. Of course, he's a handsome old man, I will say that.

JEFF: Better looking than me?

EVE: I'm afraid so.

JEFF: But that's just the outward shell.

EVE: Oh, I agree with you. I agree completely. An old, old handsome man. Can you think of anything more boring than an old, old handsome man? *(After a moment)* What time is it?

THE ROAD NOT TAKEN

JEFF: You mean actual time? It's...let me see...ten thirty five, no, no, no. It's ten thirty six going on ten thirty seven. Why?

EVE: I'm usually in bed by ten?

JEFF: Really?

EVE: Not asleep.

JEFF : What then?

EVE: I'm usually holding a book.

JEFF: *(Consolingly)* Ohhhhhh.

EVE: A boring book, one that will make me sleepy.

JEFF: *(After a moment)* Would you like something to drink?

EVE: I think I've had enough to drink?

JEFF: Would you mind if I had a drink?

EVE: It's your stomach, and your head.

JEFF: I've got some ginger ale.

EVE: I think I'd better not.

JEFF: *(Suggestively)* What?

EVE: What did you think I meant?

JEFF: I asked you first?

EVE: You're confusing me.

131

THE ROAD NOT TAKEN

JEFF: Suppose you didn't go back...to Ohio? What then?

EVE: I've got to go back.

JEFF: Why?

EVE: I'm here on a fellowship. The university is sponsoring this trip.

JEFF: Well, you took the course, didn't you? Courses?

EVE: Well, yes.

JEFF: So there you are.

EVE: Yes, but I'm supposed to report back to them. I'm supposed to use what I've learned.

JEFF: And what have you learned?

EVE: I've learned that you are a wicked man, and that Eve is being sorely tempted.

JEFF: Am I Adam?

EVE: No, you're the snake. Or maybe you're both, both Adam and the snake. I really should go.

JEFF: Do you want to go?

EVE: No.

JEFF: Then stay. Nothing's going to happen that you don't want to happen.

EVE: May I have some wine?

THE ROAD NOT TAKEN

JEFF: You sure?

EVE: Positive.

JEFF: One wine coming up.

(HE pours a glass of wine and hands it to her.)

EVE: Now, tell me about your novel.

JEFF: What do you want to know?

EVE: What's it about?

JEFF: My family.

EVE: How interesting.

JEFF: I hope so.

EVE: How far have you gotten?

JEFF; I've completed one chapter?

EVE: May I look at it?

JEFF: Now?

EVE: Why not?

JEFF: I've never shown it to anyone.

EVE: Why?

JEFF: Because I think it's hard for people to be objective, especially people I know. The people whose opinion I value, that is. *(After a moment)* Okay. *(HE goes off and returns a moment later with the manuscript, which he hands to EVE.)* Be gentle, please. It's my first time.

EVE: Thank you.

> *(HE sits, sipping his drink. SHE opens the manuscript and starts to read, when the phone rings.)*

EVE: That's the phone.

JEFF: Yes, I know. Let it ring.

> *(The phone continues to ring. HE finally sighs, gets up and answers the phone.)*

JEFF: Hello? Yes, Don, what is it? Where are you? Where?! Okay, okay. I'll be right over. *(HE hangs up.)* I've got to go. It's Don. He's got a problem, and he needs my help.

EVE: Is it serious?

JEFF: Well, sort of. I've got to go.

EVE: Do you want me to come with you?

JEFF: No, no. And, the fact is I'll be bringing him back here.

EVE: I see.

JEFF: Damn it!

EVE: May I take this with me?

JEFF: It's my only copy.

THE ROAD NOT TAKEN

EVE: I'll guard it with my life, and I'll return it to you, first thing in the morning. *(SHE returns the manuscript into the envelope.)*

JEFF: First thing in the morning.

EVE; I promise.

JEFF; Okay. We'd better get started. I'll get a cab and drop you off first.

EVE: I hope it's not too serious.

> *(HE turns off the lights, and THEY go off as the house lights come down.)*

ACT TWO

Scene One

(Three hours later. JEFF enters, turning on the lights, followed by DON.)

DON: I need a drink.

JEFF: What would you like?

DON: Make it Scotch. I know, I know. And it does taste like medicine. Oh, hell! Make it wine. Any wine. That son-of-a-bitch!

JEFF: *(HE pours a glass of wine and hands it to DON.)* Who? *(HE pours himself a Scotch.)*

DON: That fuckin' detective. He came on to me.

JEFF: Where was this?

DON: I was coming out of this bar...

JEFF: What bar is that?

DON: This gay bar on McDougal Street.

JEFF: What were you doing in a gay bar?

DON: What does one go to a gay bar for? I was trying to pick someone up. *(HE takes a sip of the wine.)*

JEFF: A man? I'm sorry. I'm a little confused, and surprised, to say the least.

DON: I know, I know. Well, I'm afraid big brother has his little surprises.

136

THE ROAD NOT TAKEN

JEFF: How long has this been going on?

DON: You want the history of my double life?

JEFF: Well, yes.

DON: Well, Doctor, it started out... let me see. It started out back home, when Artie... I don't know if you remember Artie. Well, anyway he took a bunch of us down into the cellar and showed us what this thing between our legs was good for.

JEFF: Masturbation?

DON: Bingo. And then, when I was in the army... I was sitting in the movies, this was a movie theatre at Fort Bragg. I was sitting there in the dark, watching this movie with Audrey Hepburn, and I noticed this guy sitting next to me, moving closer and closer. Finally his leg rubs up against mine, and he ends up putting his hand where it didn't belong.

JEFF: What did you do?

DON: I didn't do anything. I was horny. I mean I was ready to go out of my mind.

JEFF: So what happened?

DON: He led me outside to the back of the theatre, and he relieved me of my burden, a burden I'd been carrying around for weeks and weeks. And, I tell you, it was really great. And I thought to myself, how really thoughtful it was for this guy to be so considerate. What a noble gesture!

JEFF: A noble gesture?!

DON: A noble gesture, to go out of his way to give pleasure to someone, a complete stranger. And then I realized, if I couldn't get a woman, there was always a substitute, and I tell you that was very reassuring. I needn't be a prisoner, a prisoner dependent on the whim of some woman. Now I know what Blanche meant when she spoke about "the kindness of strangers."

JEFF: Blanche?

DON: A Streetcar Named Desire. I never did find out how that movie ended.

JEFF: Streetcar?

DON: No, the one with Audrey Hepburn.

JEFF: Does this mean...?

DON: What? That I'm gay? That's a good question. If one dips one's toes occasionally, is one gay, or not?

JEFF: You're asking me?

DON: It was a rhetorical question. The fact the matter is, I still prefer women. There might, however, be a little detour now and then. *(HE takes a sip of the wine.)* I'm sorry I put you through all that trouble, and embarrassment. I wouldn't have called you, but I didn't have enough money on me to pay the fine.

JEFF: What were you arrested for?

DON: The term was "soliciting." And the detective lied. He said I came on to him. And he really went out of his way.

JEFF: I don't understand.

DON: What don't you understand?

THE ROAD NOT TAKEN

JEFF: Why do you need a substitute?

DON: I just can't jump into bed with a woman. It's gotta be more than that.

JEFF: And with a man?

DON: It's a physical act, pure and simple. There are times when desire becomes overwhelming, when I need some release, right then and there, so I can go about my business.

JEFF: Are you still in love with Nancy?

DON: Yes, I'm still in love with Nancy, even though she is a traitor. "Till death do us part."

JEFF: Nancy wants a family. You can't blame her for that.

DON: I can, and I do. She took a sacred oath, and she broke it.

JEFF: Well, frankly, Don, I can't say that I blame her.

DON: Whose side are you on?

JEFF: Let's face it. You are now in your thirties.

DON: Very early thirties.

JEFF: When are you going to start to make a living?

DON: When I start.

JEFF: So you're willing to give up a normal life, just to be on the stage?

DON: A normal life. What is that exactly?

THE ROAD NOT TAKEN

JEFF: Why do you shake your head?

DON: Because I feel sorry for you, that's why.

JEFF: **You** feel sorry for **me?**

DON: That's right. Because I am not deluding myself. I face the facts head on.

JEFF: And what are the facts?

DON: This business of being an artist. Yes, it helps if you have talent, but talent is not the end-all, or the be-all. Being an artist, dear boy...it's not for the weak. It's not for the squeamish. If it's not do or die, if it's not your religion, forget it.

JEFF: Theatre is your religion?

DON: That's right. It's my religion, and I am its god.

JEFF: Don, you are scaring me.

DON: When I get up on that stage, I am a god.

JEFF: You're a god?

DON: That's right. I am a god. Like the preacher says, God is in all of us. Some of us are small gods, tin gods, worthless gods. And some of us are noble gods.

JEFF: Are you sure we're not talking about vanity, about ego?

DON: Vanity? Yes, of course, vanity, and selfishness, and egotism, because we need all that for the battle.

JEFF: The battle? What battle? The battle for what?

THE ROAD NOT TAKEN

DON: If you have to ask, dear brother... I read that paper you wrote about Thomas Wolfe. You have talent. There's no doubt about that. But you're never gonna make it. You don't want to offend anybody. Good God! You're smiling. What?

JEFF: Don, you are the one with the problem, not me. (*HE sips his Scotch.*)

DON: We both have a problem, son. I'm coping with mine. (*HE takes a sip of the wine.*) How did you make out with Eve, by the way?

JEFF: What's that?

DON: Eve. That sweet little girl.

JEFF: She's not a little girl.

DON: She's a little girl. I think she needs a daddy.

JEFF: Don't we all.

DON: What's wrong with Audrey, by the way?

JEFF: Nothing's wrong with Audrey. She's not for me, that's all.

DON: Why?

JEFF: Because she wants me to be something I'm not.

DON: And what might that be?

JEFF: Her dead lover, for one thing.

DON: Oh?

THE ROAD NOT TAKEN

JEFF: He was a poet, and he died in an accident. Whether she admits it or not, she's always comparing the two of us. And, of course, I come up short. And, aside from that, she's sarcastic, she's critical, and she thinks she knows it all.

DON: Maybe she does.

JEFF: How much time did you spend with her?

DON: It doesn't take long to size someone up. I like her.

JEFF: Good. So, you go after her. Marry her. That's what she wants. *(HE sips his Scotch.)* So...what are you gonna do now? What are you gonna do with your life?

DON: Right now? I'm gonna see what's casting, and start making the rounds, and I hope you're gonna put me up until I can find a place of my own. As a matter of fact, Audrey's moving out of her apartment, and she's gonna recommend me to the landlord. Meanwhile, I'll take the sofa, if that's all right with you.

JEFF: Fine.

DON: I'll chip in for the food, of course. By the way, what do you do for a living now?

JEFF: Right now I'm working part time at this language school. I teach English to foreigners.

DON: You're teaching a class?

JEFF: No, I tutor people privately, when they need me; and the people that run the school are very supportive.

DON: You make enough to live on?

THE ROAD NOT TAKEN

JEFF: And an occasional waiter's job. What?

DON: I didn't say a thing.

JEFF: Good. I'm ready for bed. I'll get out some sheets and a pillow.

DON: Thank you.

JEFF: You're welcome.

> (*JEFF goes off to the bedroom. DON sits and sips his wine. JEFF reenters with the sheets and pillow.*)

DON: Is there a news stand nearby?

JEFF: What's that? There's one on the corner. What do you need?

DON: I thought I'd get a copy of Backstage, see what's casting. I'll be right back.

> (*DON goes off. JEFF sets down the bed clothes, sits and takes a sip of his drink. HE remains seated, lost deep in thought, as the lights come down.*)

Scene Two

(The following morning. The doorbell rings. After a moment JEFF enters from the interior and opens the door. EVE is discovered.)

JEFF: Hi. Come in, come in.

EVE: I hope I'm not disturbing you.

JEFF: No, no. Can I get you some coffee...or tea?

EVE: No, no. I'm fine. How is your brother, by the way?

JEFF: Oh, he's fine.

EVE: Was it serious?

JEFF: No, no. He got into a fight with someone, and someone called the police.

EVE: *(After a moment)* I had a lovely time last night.

JEFF: So did I.

EVE: I envy you.

JEFF: Why?

EVE: You're a free soul. You can follow your heart.

JEFF: Is that so unusual?

EVE: Where I come from, it is. I've got your manuscript.

JEFF: And.

EVE: It's very interesting. What?

THE ROAD NOT TAKEN

JEFF: You can do better than that.

EVE: Well, it does need a bit of editing, but no. It does show promise. Do you plan to continue with it?

JEFF: I'm not quite sure.

EVE: It is ambitious.

JEFF: Yes, I know.

EVE: I got a call this morning...from Brad.

JEFF: Oh?

EVE: He misses me. That's the first time he's ever said that. I mean, he's so conceited. He seems to take it for granted that I'm his...possession. I'm sure he thinks of me as an adjunct, a woman who's going to be the hostess for his distinguished circle of colleagues when he invites them all in for tea. Not that he's not an attractive man. But why does he have to be so stick-in-the-mud?

JEFF: Well, maybe you'll put some life into him.

EVE: Whether I'm willing to admit it or not, I suppose I have made a commitment. Why can't he be as charming and as much fun as you are?

JEFF: In all modesty, you'd have to look far and wide for someone to rival my charm, my wit, my sensitivity.

EVE: I know you're joking, but it just happens to be true.

JEFF: I'm flattered.

THE ROAD NOT TAKEN

EVE: At any rate, he's coming into New York for the week-end. He's actually interrupted his tennis schedule to spend some time with me.

JEFF: So, there you are. And I'm sure that once you're married you'll work your charm, just as you did with me.

EVE: I'm not quite sure exactly what happened last night, but I hope I wasn't leading you on.

JEFF: You were absolutely charming.

EVE: That's what I mean. Why can't Brad be as understanding and as sensitive as you are? *(After a moment)* Maybe...

JEFF: Maybe what?

EVE: This friend you were seeing...

JEFF: No, no, no, no, no.

EVE: Why?

JEFF: We get on each others nerves.

EVE: How long....?

JEFF: Almost two years.

EVE: Then there must have been something there.

JEFF: I thought so, at first.

EVE: What is she like?

JEFF: She's a librarian.

THE ROAD NOT TAKEN

EVE: What's wrong with that?

JEFF: She's very efficient, and she thinks she knows it all.

EVE: Two years is a long time.

JEFF: It was not quite two years.

EVE: Is she pretty? You don't want to talk about it.

JEFF: There's nothing to talk about.

EVE: I really would like you to meet Brad. Maybe you can work some of your magic, and turn him into a real human being.

JEFF: Okay.

EVE: Thank you for letting me read your work. I'll be in touch.

> *(EVE kisses him impulsively and leaves. JEFF sighs, stands lost, then opens the envelope and studies the manuscript. He proceeds to tear it into little pieces and drops the pieces into a waste basket, then sits thinking. The doorbell rings. JEFF lets it ring.)*

JEFF: Oh, go away.

> *(The doorbell rings a second time. JEFF gets up and opens the door. DON enters.)*

DON: Don't you have an extra key?

JEFF: I did.

DON: *(It takes him a second to realize what he's referring to.)* Oh. *(HE stands study JEFF)* Are you all right?

147

THE ROAD NOT TAKEN

JEFF: I'm perfectly fine!!

DON Uh, oh! Tell Daddy.

JEFF: I don't think Daddy's in any position to give advice to anyone.

DON: Watch your tongue, dear boy. I'm older than you are.

JEFF: Are you, really? Seriously. What are you gonna do with your life?

DON: You asked me that.

JEFF: I'm asking you again. What are you gonna do with your life?

DON: Well, specifically...

JEFF: Specifically!

DON: This morning I went to an Equity call.

JEFF: An Equity call? You're not even a union member.

DON: I'm aware of that. Sometimes, however, when someone doesn't show up, or at the end of the call, if there's still time, I can get to read.

JEFF: I see.

DON: And this afternoon there are two Equity calls.

JEFF: So you're going to sit around and wait to see if you'll get to read. Is that it?

DON: Bingo!

THE ROAD NOT TAKEN

JEFF: Okay. Suppose you get to read, and you get hired, and you're an Equity member. What happens when the Equity show closes? What happens then?

DON: Oh, ye of little faith.

JEFF: I'm serious, Don. Is this the way you're gonna spend your life?

DON: You're beginning to sound like Mother. You thought I had talent, didn't you?

JEFF: Am I gonna give you a job? Am I a producer?

DON: No, Jeff, you're not a producer. What are you? You tell me.

JEFF: We're talking about you. Okay, okay. If that's the kind of life you want to lead, I'm happy for you.

DON: Of course, I want more. As a matter of fact, it's kind of ironic. The reason I lost my wife is because she wanted a family, she wanted children, and I was petrified at the very thought. And now, recently, I've begun to think, I really would like to have a family. I'd like to have a son, and I will, eventually.

JEFF: Eventually?

DON: Rome wasn't built in a day.

JEFF: Where do you get these brilliant observations? I mean it, Don. Let's face it. You may never make a living as an actor. What happens then?

DON: If I don't make it?

JEFF: Yes. What happens then?

THE ROAD NOT TAKEN

DON: I can say that I tried. How's the lady Eve, by the way?

JEFF: What's that? The lady Eve has left the garden of Eden.

DON: Oh? Where has she gone?

JEFF: She's gone back to her fiancee, who really isn't her fiance, but actually he is her fiancee.

DON: Maybe you ought to give Audrey a second thought.

JEFF: Is that your advice?

DON: Take it or leave it.

JEFF: Thank you.

DON: I'm gonna take a nap, if you don't mind. I didn't get any sleep last night.

JEFF: Go right ahead.

  (*DON starts off.*)

JEFF: Incidentally...

DON: Yes? I'm waiting.

JEFF: It might interest you to know that I've destroyed the first chapter of my novel.

DON: Meaning what?

JEFF: Meaning I've destroyed the first chapter of my novel.

DON: Congratulations...I think.

THE ROAD NOT TAKEN

(DON goes off. JEFF pours himself a drink and sits on the sofa nursing it. The phone rings. After the third ring HE answers it.)

JEFF: Hello? Yes, I'm home. If you like.

(HE hangs up, returns to his drink and the sofa. After a moment the doorbell rings. JEFF gets up and opens the door. AUDREY enters.)

JEFF: That was quick.

AUDREY: I live upstairs. Remember?

JEFF: What are you doing home at this hour?

AUDREY: It's Saturday, in case you've forgotten.

JEFF: What?

AUDREY: You usually don't start till cocktail hour. Shall we start?

JEFF: What's that?

AUDREY: We were going to sort things out, remember? Decide what things are yours, and what things are mine. If this is a bad time...

JEFF: No, no, no. We might as well get it over with.

AUDREY: Before we become a zombie? Sorry. Shall we start with the records?

JEFF: If you like?

THE ROAD NOT TAKEN

AUDREY: Let's see. *(SHE starts separating the records.)*The operas are mine.

JEFF: And you're welcome to them.

AUDREY: The Beethoven...

JEFF: The seventh symphony is mine. You bought it for my birthday.

AUDREY: So I did. Well, you can have all the Beethoven. The Glenn Miller, the Harry James....

JEFF: The Harry James is mine, and so is the Glenn Miller.

AUDREY: Okay, okay.

JEFF: And the Carmina Burana.

AUDREY: I bought the Carmina Burana. I was the one that told you about it.

JEFF: And I went out and bought it.

AUDREY: All right. You can have the Carmina Burana.

JEFF: Oh, look. Take whatever you like. I don't care.

AUDREY: Do you want to do this now, or don't you?

JEFF: Yes, yes. Let's get it over with.

AUDREY: Okay. Let's start on the books. I bought you the signed copy of Look Homeward, Angel.

JEFF: What really pisses me off...

THE ROAD NOT TAKEN

AUDREY: What?

JEFF: You're always comparing me to Paul. Paul wrote this, and Paul wrote that. How do you think that makes me feel?

AUDREY: I'm sorry. I was in love with him, and he was a talented man.

JEFF: And he's dead. I'm sorry, but those are the facts.

AUDREY: You're right. You're absolutely right. It was inconsiderate of me; it was insensitive.

JEFF: Do you still see that cousin of yours, the one that owns that ad agency?

AUDREY: Jeremy? I had lunch with him yesterday. As a matter of fact, he asked about you. He still talks about that paper you wrote about Thomas Wolfe. Why do you ask?

JEFF: I just wondered. Huckleberry Finn is yours, and so is Ulysses. Crime And Punishment is mine, and so is The Brothers Karamazov. Alice In Wonderland is yours. And so is the dictionary.

AUDREY: You can have the dictionary.

JEFF: Thank you. It might interest you to know...I've destroyed the first chapter of my novel.

AUDREY: I never knew there was a first chapter.

JEFF: Well, there was.

AUDREY: What about the other chapters?

THE ROAD NOT TAKEN

JEFF: There was only one chapter.

AUDREY: You do have talent.

JEFF: I know I have talent. There are other things that I don't have.

AUDREY: Like what?

JEFF: What difference does it make? What do you think of my brother?

AUDREY: He's charming. As a matter of fact, the two of you are very much alike.

JEFF: You think so?

AUDREY: Don't you?

JEFF: It's amazing. You can know someone all your life, and then you find out that you don't know them at all.

AUDREY: You always spoke so highly of him.

JEFF: He was my childhood idol, I suppose.

AUDREY: And now?

JEFF: I'm no longer a child.

AUDREY: Is that bad?

JEFF: Jeremy offered me a job, you know.

AUDREY: Yes, I know.

JEFF: That was months ago. Do you think that offer still holds good?

AUDREY: I can't speak for Jeremy, but I know he thinks a lot of you.

JEFF: Why have you suddenly decided to move to a larger apartment? You seemed perfectly content where you were. Have you suddenly found a new romance?

AUDREY: No.

JEFF: Then why are you moving?

AUDREY: The Blackwells are moving out. The apartment's going to be vacant. Rents are going up, and it would be a shame to let it go.

JEFF: Why?

AUDREY: Because.

JEFF: Because why?

AUDREY: Because my apartment is almost as small as yours; and, because...who knows what the future may bring? And, if you must know, I made these arrangements months ago, when the Blackwells said they were looking for another apartment.

JEFF: I see. Well, you certainly are the efficient one.

AUDREY: So you've said, time and time again. And I don't happen to think it's anything to be ashamed of.

JEFF: I never said that it was.

THE ROAD NOT TAKEN

AUDREY: You certainly make it sound like it was.

JEFF: Oh, look. Can't we have a civil conversation without all these snide remarks? Shall we continue with the books?

AUDREY: Oh, fuck the books!

JEFF: You're not crying, are you?

AUDREY: No. I'm too efficient to cry.

JEFF: Oh, look. I've been difficult, I know. But I've been going through some hard times...finding myself. And please, don't say I didn't know you were lost.

AUDREY: I wasn't going to say a thing.

JEFF: We are right for each other, Audrey.

AUDREY: You think so?

JEFF: Don't you?

AUDREY: I used to thinks so. I used to think that we might make a go of it. That was until we got to know one another, and then it was obvious that we lived on two different planets.

JEFF: Well, it appears that you're moving to a new apartment, and I'm moving to another planet. I'm hoping that Jeremy might give me a job.

AUDREY: While you work on your novel?

JEFF: The Carter family has only one so-called artist now, God help him.

THE ROAD NOT TAKEN

AUDREY: What brought about this sudden change?

JEFF: I think that in any relationship there are certain areas...

AUDREY: Okay, okay. I think we've done enough for today. I'll take these records up.

JEFF: Why don't you leave them here, and wait until you've moved into your new apartment?

AUDREY: I suppose I could do that. I'll just put them aside. Maybe we can finish up on the books tomorrow, if you can find the time. Well, I guess that's it. I'm sure you have things to do, and so do I.

JEFF: Yes. Yes, of course.

AUDREY: Take care.

JEFF: You, too.

    (AUDREY starts for the door.)

JEFF: Audrey...?

AUDREY: Yes?

JEFF: Nothing.

    (AUDREY hesitates for a moment and then goes off. JEFF sits, picks up his drink, and sets it down. HE sits irresolutely on the edge of the sofa, then rises, paces about, then goes to the phone. HE hesitates, plucks up his courage, picks up the phone and dials.)

THE ROAD NOT TAKEN

JEFF: Hi. It's me. Would you be interested in taking in the Saint Genaro Festival? Yes, now. Okay. I'll meet you downstairs.

(JEFF places his glass on the bar. HE runs off to the bedroom and reenters, getting into a sports jacket. HE takes a comb out of his pocket and runs it through his hair, then starts off as the lights come down and festival music is heard.)

CHOICES
A Comedy

CAST OF CHARACTERS

Henri Prideaux

Claudette Duval Prideaux

Sacha Prideaux

Danielle Moray

SCENE
Paris
The rehearsal room in Le Theatre Moderne.

TIME
The nineteen thirties.

ACT ONE

(The rehearsal room. The stage right door leads to the theatre. The stage left door leads to the Prideaux living quarters. It's Autumn. Early afternoon. CLAUDETTE, a slim, lovely woman in her late fifties, enters from the theatre, followed by her son, SACHA, a pleasant looking young man of twenty-one, and HENRI, an imposing figure of a man of sixty.)

CLAUDETTE: That was a lovely ceremony. How long has it been now?

HENRI: Fifteen years.

CLAUDETTE: Fifteen years. I can't believe it.

HENRI: *(Sarcastically. He's obviously annoyed about something.)* How time flies. *(Impatiently)* Are you going to pour, or shall I?

SACHA: Why don't I do the pouring for a change? *(HE opens the liquor cabinet and pours three glasses of cognac.)*

HENRI: It's all so depressing.

CLAUDETTE: *(Trying to control her anger)* You know, my dear.... If I remember correctly, the memorial was your idea to begin with.

HENRI: I'm aware of that. I never meant, however, for it to become a meaningless ritual. As if we needed to be reminded that a great man of the theatre has left us. Papa *(pronounced paPAH)* despised sentimentality.

SACHA: I remember him as a sweet, gentle man.

HENRI: You were five years old. What do you remember?

CHOICES

SACHA: He used to tell me stories.

HENRI: Do you remember how he looked forward to seeing you on the stage, all three of us, working together? Do you remember that?

SACHA: *(HE hands HENRI a glass of cognac.)* No. *(HE hands CLAUDETTE a glass of cognac.)*

CLAUDETTE: Thank you, dear.

HENRI: It's a family tradition, he said. And he set the bar. Camille opposite Bernhardt, sharing her triumph in The Eaglet. Phedre, opposite the immortal Rachel. The Misanthrope. The School For Wives. I'm boring you.

SACHA: You do have a habit of repeating yourself.

CLAUDETTE: Sacha!

SACHA: I loved Papa Maurice, but he was not a saint. I propose a toast, a toast to a gentleman who lived life to the fullest. To Papa Maurice!

CLAUDETTE: To Papa Maurice.

(THEY drink.)

HENRI: Obviously your time in England has really paid off.

SACHA: I'm sorry, Papa. I don't mean to be impertinent, but sometimes you do go on. We had a very special relationship, Papa Maurice and I, and I remember him as a jolly man, with a wonderful, resounding laugh, and a wicked twinkle in his eye.

CLAUDETTE: He adored you, Sacha.

161

CHOICES

HENRI: Much good it did him.

SACHA: Papa, I've interrupted my studies. I've agreed to work with you, in your new play, in a role, I've been continually reminded, was written especially for me.

HENRI: My cup runneth over.

CLAUDETTE: Henri, Sacha's here. What more do you want?

HENRI: I want a son. That's what I want.

SACHA: No, Papa, that's not what you want. What you want is someone to carry on what you call your legacy. However, if I remember correctly, Papa Maurice had the very same complaint about you. "I don't want a flibbertigibbet. a writer of boulevard comedies, an actor of all style and little substance."

HENRI: You remember all that, do you, even though you were five years old.

SACHA: No, Papa. I'm quoting you.

HENRI: All right, so we had our differences. But did I desert him? Did I run off to that island inhabited by people with ice in their veins?

CLAUDETTE: Henri, the boy is willing to work with you.

HENRI: I don't want someone who's willing to work with me. I have my pick of every actor in Paris. Why should I settle for someone who's willing to work with me?

SACHA: Oh, for God's sake, Papa, No tears, please!

(*SACHA approaches HENRI and they embrace.*)

162

CHOICES

HENRI: Oh, my dear, dear boy, if only you knew the dreams I had for you, for us, working as a team, together. And it's not only that. As you well know, Papa turned up his nose at my comedies, my "cotton candy" he called them. He wanted me to write a tragedy, a tragedy especially for him and, selfish brute that I was, I refused. "Its not my style," I said. And now, now I've finally found my tragic voice. The Kingdom By The Sea is my first attempt at a tragedy, a classical tragedy to rival Corneille, to rival Racine. It may be too late for Papa Maurice, but now, you and I, the two of us, will appear together, for the very first time in something completely new.

SACHA: I'm looking forward to it, Papa. I really am.

CLAUDETTE: Henri...

HENRI: What were those lines from Chekhov? Trepleff, the young playwright. "We need new forms..."

CLAUDETTE: Henri...

HENRI: "And if we can't have them, it's better to have nothing at all." Yes? What is it?

CLAUDETTE: The new ingenue. She's been waiting very patiently.

SACHA: New ingenue?

CLAUDETTE: Dora's pregnant.

HENRI: I'll see her shortly. I've made some changes in the script. They're minor ones, but I want to point them out. We'll go into my study.

> (CLAUDETTE sighs, shakes her head and goes off to the theatre.)

163

CHOICES

HENRI: Nothing is written in stone. If there's something that bothers you...

(HENRI places his arm around SACHA's shoulder and THEY go off to the living quarters. A moment later CLAUDETTE enters with DANIELLE, a pretty young lady in her twenties.)

CLAUDETTE: I'm sorry. It's been such a hectic day.

DANIELLE: Oh, that's quite all right. It's been a great privilege to attend the memorial. Maurice Prideaux was such a great artist.

CLAUDETTE: You're so young, my dear. You couldn't possibly have seen Maurice Prideaux.

DANIELLE: I never saw him in person, but my family often spoke about him; and I've read so much about him,

CLAUDETTE: Please, have a seat.

DANIELLE: Thank you.

(THEY sit.)

CLAUDETTE: Tell me, my dear, how long have you been married?

DANIELLE: I beg your pardon?

CLAUDETTE: You've removed the ring, I see, but there are still some telltale signs.

DANIELLE: May I be frank?

CLAUDETTE: Please.

CHOICES

DANIELLE: When I met Monsieur Prideaux, he spoke rather bitterly about Mademoiselle LaMarr's pregnancy and how, if one is serious, ones private life must not interfere with ones career.

CLAUDETTE: So you thought it might be wise to let him to believe that you were single.

DANIELLE: When I removed my gloves, I carefully removed my wedding ring as well, and I noticed that Monsieur's eyes went directly to my wedding ring finger, and he did seem pleased. I do hope my marriage won't stand in my way.

CLAUDETTE: Your secret is safe with me.

DANIELLE: Thank you. I so looked forward to working with your company, and especially with you, Madame. But now it appears that you won't be appearing in Monsieur's new play.

CLAUDETTE: Apparently, since my husband saw fit to write only one female role, and an ingenue at that. So, tell me, how long have you been married?

DANIELLE: One year.

CLAUDETTE: The first year. Ah, yes! Then you're still on your honeymoon.

DANIELLE: Hardly. My husband's studying to be a doctor. At present, he's serving an internship, and his hours are so erratic. In addition to that, there's my performance schedule in the theatre. It makes for a rather hectic domestic life. But we love each other so. Nothing can ever come between us.

CLAUDETTE: Ah, yes.

CHOICES

DANIELLE: Oh, I knew you'd understand. You and monsieur, your romance is legendary. I often wondered...

CLAUDETTE: What?

DANIELLE: Your secret. After all these years... How does one hold on to a man as fascinating as Monsieur, a man with so many opportunities?

CLAUDETTE: Keep your figure, my dear. A woman can be stupid. A woman can be foolish, but a woman should never grow fat.

DANIELLE: I shall keep that in mind.

CLAUDETTE: Have you read the new play?

DANIELLE: Oh yes.

CLAUDETTE: And...

DANIELLE: It's so unusual.

CLAUDETTE: A tragedy, yes. It's a bit of a change for you, as well as my husband.

DANIELLE: Oh, yes. A departure from light comedy. That's what makes it so exciting. In addition to that, the opportunity to appear on the same stage opposite Henri Prideaux! Even Jacques, my husband, is impressed, and he's always so matter-of-fact; which is understandable, of course. When one deals daily with life and death, the theatre seems so frivolous.

CLAUDETTE: Does he approve of your career?

CHOICES

DANIELLE: He has no say in the matter, since what he earns doesn't even pay the rent.

CLAUDETTE: Ah, yes. There's always a price to be paid. I wanted more children, but three mouths to feed, and a theatre to run... Life is full of choices, my dear, and who's to say which is the wisest?

DANIELLE: Has the role of the son been cast?

CLAUDETTE: Oh, yes. Our son, Sacha, will be making his debut.

DANIELLE: Oh? I thought your son was at a university in Great Britain.

CLAUDETTE: He's taken a leave of absence.

DANIELLE: Oh? He's joined the company,

CLAUDETTE: Yes, well...as far as that's concerned, that remains to be seen.

(HENRI enters.)

HENRI: Ah, you're here.

(DANIELLE rises.)

HENRI: Sit, sit.

CLAUDETTE: I'd better see how our dinner's progressing.

HENRI: Perhaps Mademoiselle Moray would care to join us for dinner.

CLAUDETTE: Mademoiselle Moray may have made other plans. Besides, Marie is preparing a dinner for three.

CHOICES

HENRI: The master has spoken. You see, my dear, I may be in charge of our theatre. Madame, however, is in charge of our life.

CLAUDETTE: Poor darling.

HENRI: And, incidentally, Sacha's room hasn't been readied for him.

CLAUDETTE: Yes, I know. Excuse me. *(SHE goes off.)*

HENRI: *(HE sits with a sigh.)* Thank God there's no performance tonight. What was it that Englishman....Bernard Shaw...once said? "Youth is wasted on the young."

DANIELLE: With age comes wisdom, does it not?

HENRI: I'll gladly trade that phantom wisdom for the vigor of youth, and those youthful dreams.

DANIELLE: Surely, Monsieur, all your dreams have come true.

HENRI: Some of them, oh yes.

DANIELLE: To be thought of as one of our finest actors.

HENRI: Alongside the legendary Jean Coquelin? Alongside Louis Jouvet? Yes, well, who's to say?

DANIELLE: And as a playwright.

HENRI: So, you've read the play, my first tragedy.

DANIELLE: Oh, yes, and I think the role of Therese is an absolutely magnificent creation. It's a gift to an actress, and I feel so honored to be chosen.

CHOICES

HENRI: You know, of course, that our theatre operates on a very limited budget. People seem to think, "Oh, Prideaux! Look at those costumes. Look at those sets." Our productions are lavish, it's true; but the money has got to come from somewhere. So if you expect to get rich working for us....

DANIELLE: Oh no, Monsieur. I don't expect to get rich.

HENRI: My wife and I are dedicated artists, and we expect those who work with us to devote the same passion that we demand of ourselves.

DANIELLE: I'm a serious artist, Monsieur.

HENRI: I'm sure you are. And you will find, my dear, as the years go by, that's where one finds the greatest joy in life. Work is what keeps one young. Work is what makes life worth living.

DANIELLE: Oh, I quite agree.

HENRI: *(After a moment)* So...any questions?

DANIELLE: I can think of none at the moment.

HENRI: Good. I'll introduce you now to Monsieur Bertrand, our business manager. *(HE rises.)* Come along.

> *(DANIELLE rises and THEY start towards the theatre, when SACHA enters from the living quarters.)*

SACHA: Oh, I beg your pardon. I was looking for Mama. (Pronounced maMAH) *(HE starts to leave.)*

HENRI: No, no. Stay. I'd like you to meet our leading lady. Danielle Moray this is Sacha Prideaux. You're going to see a lot of one another.

169

CHOICES

SACHA: Charmed.

DANIELLE: Likewise.

(SHE extends her hand and HE kisses it.)

HENRI: *(To DANIELLE)* Shall we go? *(To SACHA)* We were just about to arrange Danielle's contract. *(To DANIELLE)* Come along. *(To SACHA)* Your mother is seeing to your room.

SACHA: Thank you.

(HENRI nods at DANIELLE and THEY go off to the theatre. SACHA sits with a sigh. CLAUDETTE enters.)

CLAUDETTE: I'm sorry about the room, dear.

SACHA: All those books, all those manuscripts. I was afraid to touch anything.

CLAUDETTE: I know. I've been so busy. *(SHE sits beside SACHA.)* So. We've missed you.

SACHA: I've missed you, too.

CLAUDETTE: Yes, I'm sure you have.

SACHA: In spite of the fact that you've ruined my life.

CLAUDETTE: Oh? And how, pray tell, is that?

SACHA: Every girl I meet I ask myself, "Is she as pretty as Mama? Is she as clever as Mama?"

CLAUDETTE: Well, you've learned one thing from your father.

CHOICES

SACHA: And what might that be?

CLAUDETTE: How to flatter a woman. So, how does it feel to be back home? Oh, dear.

SACHA: What?

CLAUDETTE: That martyred look.

SACHA: You blackmailed me. Yes, blackmailed.

CLAUDETTE: Sacha, I just presented the facts. Your father's come to realize he's not as vigorous as he once was, and it frightens him. We need you here...at least for now. Is that too much to ask?

SACHA: He expects me to stay on. He expects me to join the company.

CLAUDETTE: I know what he expects.

SACHA: He has the theatre in his blood, and he's convinced himself that it's my duty to follow in his footsteps. The fact of the matter is, I have a mind of my own.

CLAUDETTE: Sacha, you're here for my sake as well as his.

SACHA: What do you want me to do?

CLAUDETTE: I want you to do the best you can, while you're here. What do you think of the play?

SACHA: It's depressing. People will come to see a Prideaux play expecting to be amused. As a matter of fact, I think we may be getting laughs all right, in all the wrong places.

CLAUDETTE: It's different, of course, and it is a challenge. But we do have our following. In addition to that, this is an occasion, the young Prideaux at his father's side. They'll come out of curiosity, out of sentiment perhaps. As a matter of fact, for all we know, we may have a great success on our hands.

SACHA: It would just be my luck.

CLAUDETTE: Stop it! Do you hear me? Stop it! All I hear from you is what you don't want. You don't want to be an actor. You don't want to be a playwright. What **do** you want to do?

SACHA: I'm interested in history. I'm interested in philosophy.

CLAUDETTE: And how do you plan to support yourself?

SACHA: I don't know. Maybe I'll teach. Maybe I'll write.

CLAUDETTE: Teach what? Write what?

SACHA: Philosophical history. Historical philosophy. I don't know. Maybe I'll be another Descartes.

(*HENRI enters.*)

HENRI: All this fuss because your room isn't ready?

CLAUDETTE: Nobody's making a fuss.

SACHA: I was afraid of disturbing things. I'll take care of it myself. I'll just make two piles. One pile of all the manuscripts, and another of all those documents. I'll be very careful. I promise.

(*SACHA goes off to the living quarters. HENRI sits with a sigh.*)

CLAUDETTE: You look tired.

172

CHOICES

HENRI: I didn't sleep well last night.

CLAUDETTE: Yes, I know.

HENRI: He's changed.

CLAUDETTE: You think so?

HENRI: He's not a boy any longer Am I asking too much? Tell me. Am I being unreasonable? I was only too happy to work with my father. The fact of the matter is I know my son better he knows himself. Whether he's aware of it or not, the theatre's in his blood. Once he steps out on that stage, once he feels that electricity passing from him to the darkness out there; once he experiences the thrill of moving an audience, moving them to laughter, moving them to tears, that's when he'll be mine again. You wait and see. Oh, you think you're so clever with that sweet, innocent madonna look.

CLAUDETTE: A madonna am I?

HENRI: A lascivious madonna. I don't know what you're up to.

CLAUDETTE: Why should I be up to something? I'm perfectly content.

(HE eyes her skeptically.)

CLAUDETTE: I've been happily married for twenty five years. I've been doing the work I love for even longer. We're both in reasonably good health, and we've got a beautiful son.

HENRI: You're such a liar.

CLAUDETTE: I don't know what you're talking about.

CHOICES

HENRI: For one thing, this is the first time in almost ten years you will not be appearing alongside me in one of my plays.

CLAUDETTE: I could use a vacation.

HENRI: Lie number two.

CLAUDETTE: I'm a comedienne. Kingdom By The Sea is not my cup of tea.

HENRI: You've said nothing about what you think of the piece.

CLAUDETTE: As you yourself have said, "My plays are always a work in progress."

HENRI: *(After a moment)* You're not jealous, are you?

CLAUDETTE: Jealous?

HENRI: Of our new ingenue?

CLAUDETTE: Have I reason to be?

HENRI: You did not approve of her.

CLAUDETTE: She's a delightful actress, but I think you've made a mistake. The role of Therese is not an ingenue role. The girl you wrote may be young in years, but she's tough. She's suffered.

HENRI: You think you could play the role?

CLAUDETTE: Ten years ago, yes. Well, maybe twelve. You had Dora in mind when you wrote that role, and I think she would have brought something very special.

HENRI: In the condition she's in?

CHOICES

CLAUDETTE: She's due in two months. You could have waited.

HENRI: For the past ten years, the season has always opened with a play by Henri Prideaux. And besides, I think you're wrong about the girl. And she's a perfect match for Sacha, a perfect match, in more ways then one. Don't you think?

CLAUDETTE: Oh, yes. They make a handsome couple.

HENRI: And who knows? Who knows what the future may hold? I want you to sit in on rehearsals. As a matter of fact, I'd like you to take charge.

CLAUDETTE: Oh?

HENRI: You've done it before, and I do feel a little uneasy.

CLAUDETTE: If that's what you want. *(SHE rises.)*

HENRI: Where are you going?

CLAUDETTE: I'd better take charge of Sacha's room. There are all sorts of important papers, and I don't want them thrown about. I'll let you know when dinner's ready. Sit.

> *(SHE places a kiss on the top of his head and goes off. HENRI sighs, and sits thoughtfully as the lights come down.)*

Scene Two

(Two days later. Ten in the morning. SACHA is seated, studying his script. DANIELLE, carrying a briefcase, enters from the theatre.)

DANIELLE: I'm not late, am I?

SACHA: No, no. You're just in time.

DANIELLE: The traffic was awful. And I started out very early. Are you nervous? No, of course not. As far as you're concerned, this is just another rehearsal.

SACHA: Not exactly.

DANIELLE: What was it like, growing up with Henri Prideaux as your father, and Claudette Duval as your mother?

SACHA: They were my parents.

DANIELLE: You must have been aware of the fact that they were someone special. I grew up on a farm, in the provinces. I wanted to become a movie star, like Greta Garbo, and my parents were not too happy about my becoming an actress; my father, that is. He's a school teacher, and very proper. My mother was pleased, however. She loves the theatre. Well, the cinema really. Maurice Chevalier, Jean Gabin, Dannielle Darrieux. She keeps hoping that someone from some big studio in America will come to see me perform, and whisk me away to Hollywood.

SACHA: And you? What do you hope?

DANIELLE: My hope has come true. One of them, at any rate. To work with your parents in their theatre.

SACHA: You don't want to become a film star?

CHOICES

DANIELLE: I want to keep working. And, so far, I've been lucky. Oh, I don't fool myself. It helps to be pretty. But I do work hard, and I'm not silly, like some girls I know. I like to work with serious artists. That's why I'm so excited to be working on this play. I think it's a masterpiece. Don't you? And I think your father is highly underrated. Just because he writes comedies... Well, when the critic comes to see this play, they will certainly change their tune. Don't you think?

SACHA: Quite possibly.

DANIELLE: *(After a moment)* What do you think?

SACHA: About what?

DANIELLE: About the play

SACHA: It's an interesting departure.

DANIELLE: That's all?

SACHA: I could never be objective. I know the playwright too well. I'm concentrating on the role, and it happens to be a role I feel comfortable with.

DANIELLE: What do you think of Therese?

SACHA: She's fascinating.

DANIELLE: You don't think she's too...

SACHA: Too what?

DANIELLE: Too...dramatic.

SACHA: You mean...she does things for effect?

CHOICES

DANIELLE: No. Not deliberately.

SACHA: She's strong.

DANIELLE: Like a man?

SACHA: You think men have a monopoly on strength?

DANIELLE: Do you think she's sympathetic?

SACHA: She's admirable.

DANIELLE: You think so?

SACHA: Don't you?

DANIELLE: I should be discussing this with the playwright.

SACHA: When he arrives.

DANIELLE: *(After a moment)* Do you think she's in love with the father...or the son?

SACHA: I don't think she's in love with either of them.

DANIELLE: You think she's cold?

SACHA: Not necessarily.

DANIELLE: I'm sorry. I'm very nervous.

SACHA: That's a good sign.

DANIELLE: I'll bet you'd make a wonderful director.

SACHA: Why do you say that?

CHOICES

DANIELLE: You seem so...so...

SACHA: So what?

DANIELLE: So down to earth.

SACHA: Acting, Danielle, is not exactly brain surgery. I know some very stupid actors who happen to be very talented. And some very intelligent actors who are actually rather boring.

DANIELLE: Where would I fit in, do you think?

SACHA: I haven't quite decided.

DANIELLE: I talk too much, I know.

SACHA: If it makes you feel any better, you have my blessing.

DANIELLE: Thank you.

> (THEY sit silently, each lost in their private thoughts. After a moment CLAUDETTE enters from the theatre.)

CLAUDETTE: I'm sorry. There seems to be a slight disagreement between the producer and the set designer.

SACHA: What's the problem?

CLAUDETTE: The producer wants a stylized set.

SACHA: And Etienne?

CLAUDETTE: A naturalistic set.

SACHA: I thought he was going to find a new set designer.

CHOICES

CLAUDETTE: He couldn't find the right one.

(HENRI enters from the theatre.)

HENRI: Sorry to keep you waiting. I was hoping to have a set design to display but, unfortunately, we've run into some problems.

CLAUDETTE: It's just as well. Before we start to read, before we start to discuss the play, I think it's important, first of all, for us to get to know one another. I'd like to start out with a couple of questions.

HENRI: Oh?

CLAUDETTE: Question number one. What was your most satisfying theatrical experience? Take your time. Henri, why don't we start out you.

HENRI: Well, let me see.

CLAUDETTE: Take your time. Your most satisfying theatrical experience.

HENRI: Well, actually, my most satisfying experience in the theatre would need sort of a prologue.

CLAUDETTE: We're listening. Go on.

HENRI: Well, I was twenty one when I was cast by my father in a curtain-raiser, La Bonne Helene by Lemaitre. I wore a very ornate costume, and I wanted to have a picture of myself in the costume, so in between the matinee and evening performance, I sneaked out of the theatre in my costume, which was against the rules, and took a taxi to my friend's studio on the other side of town, and I arrived at the theatre just in time to make my entrance. The leading lady, complimenting me on my elegant appearance,

180

CHOICES

could hardly keep a straight face. She finally burst out laughing, and so did the rest of the cast, and suddenly I realized that I'd left my wig and my elegant hat in the taxi.

DANIELLE: Oh dear.

HENRI: Yes. Well, my father summoned me into his office. I would have to pay a fine, he said, of one hundred francs...for being late and for losing an expensive hat. "That's a little much," I said. "Take it or leave it," he said. I left it, and the company, and my father and I never spoke for almost six years.

DANIELLE: Oh, how awful.

HENRI: That was the prologue. Six years later. I was appearing, quite successfully, in my comedy, The Lady In Question, when word came back that my father was in the audience.

DANIELLE: Oh my.

HENRI: Oh, yes. I was a nervous wreck. After the performance Papa came back stage. "You were quite good," he said. And then he said, "I would like you to write a play for me, a comedy."

DANIELLE: You must have been pleased.

HENRI: Yes, well, strangely enough, for quite some time, I'd been thinking about a comedy with my father in mind for the leading role. I wrote the play, he thought it was clever, and we went into rehearsal. Opening night was a triumph. The applause went on for almost ten minutes. And then there was a call for "Author, author

DANIELLE: How wonderful!

HENRI: My father stepped forward and held up his hand. "I have been privileged." he said, "to introduce an author from time to time, but nothing has given me more pleasure than to present this gifted playwright to you." I came on stage. My father and I embraced, and we were both in tears.

DANIELLE: Ohhh.

HENRI: And that was the most memorable moment in my career...in my life, I might say.

(DANIELLE and SACHA applaud.)

HENRI: Except, of course, for my wedding day.

CLAUDETTE: Yes, of course. Danielle, what was your most satisfying theatrical experience.

DANIELLE: Let me see. I was hired by this provincial theatre for a production of The Bourgeois Gentilhomme. I played the daughter and I was very well received, and the producer was very pleased. They were sending out a first class tour of The Misanthrope and I was cast as Celimene.

SACHA: Good for you!

DANIELLE: I was in heaven. The producer came to see our first performance and, believe it or not, he wanted me replaced.

SACHA: Good lord! Why? I thought he was pleased with your work.

DANIELLE: So did I. Apparently I was too weak. I had no get up and go. The stage manager, however, was very sympathecic. He persuaded the producer to give me another chance.

HENRI: Lucky for you

CHOICES

DANIELLE: Yes, well, the producer agreed to come back the following week, and he would make up his mind. The stage manager then told me to take center stage, and to speak up. I did the best that I could.

HENRI: And?

DANIELLE: Two weeks later the producer came back. "Well," he said, "she's still not an ideal Celimene, but, I suppose, she'll do."

(SACHA and HENRI applaud.)

DANIELLE: Oh, yes. But, my real triumph came later. In every single review I was hightly praised. I remember...in one review in particular the critic wrote, "Danielle Moray as Celimene sparkled wittily,and added a much needed spirit to an otherwise pedestrian production."

(HENRI and SACHA applaud loudly.)

SACHA: Brava! That showed him.

HENRI: Well done!

CLAUDETTE: Sacha?

SACHA: Well, my experience on stage, as you well know has been very limited.

CLAUDETTE: Go on.

SACHA: Well, I suppose my most satisfying theatrical experience took place when I was in the audience. I was taken by Papa Maurice to this magnificent theatre. I must have been about three or so. The curtain went up, and there was this strange room. Papa come into this strange room with a strange lady. Then Mama came into the room with some strange man. And then Papa and Mama began to quarrel and throw things at each other, and then finally they kissed, and they seemed to be very happy, and that made me happy, too.

(Applause)

DANIELLE: You didn't realize they were performing?

SACHA: I did wonder why they were in this strange house, until Papa Maurice explained that this was a game they played to make money to pay for our food and our clothes. I thought that was a rather funny way of making money.

CLAUDETTE: And so it is. One final question. Why did you decide to become an actor? Henri?

HENRI: Well, actually I avoided the theatre at first. I was good at sketching and I looked into art as a career That led nowhere, I toyed with journalism. That led nowhere. Finally I approached Papa Maurice, and told him that I was going to be an actor. I expected to be welcomed with open arms.

SACHA: And what did he say?

HENRI: All he said was, "Fine. Good luck."

SACHA: Really?

HENRI: Yes, really. And actually, he did me a favor. Because that was when I realized, that that what was what I really wanted to do. I really wanted to be an actor.

(Applause)

HENRI: And, so here I am!

CHOICES

(Applause)

CLAUDETTE: Danielle?

DANIELLE: I was terribly shy, and there was an acting club in our school and, in order to overcome my shyness, I joined the club and, of course, I was hooked.

(Applause)

CLAUDETTE: Sacha?

SACHA: I haven't decided to become an actor.

(There is a moment of silence.)

CLAUDETTE: Well, since we started late, and it's almost time for lunch, this might be a good time to take a break.

HENRI: What's that? Yes. Yes, of course.

CLAUDETTE: The table in the dining room's all set. Why don't you go right in. Sacha, why don't you lead the way.

SACHA: *(HE turns to DANIELLE and holds out his arm.)* May I?

(DANIELLE takes SACHA's arm and THEY go off.)

CLAUDETTE: You don't want him to lie, do you?

HENRI: At this point I couldn't care less.

(HENRI strides off. CLAUDETTE shrugs, shakes her head and follows him off as the lights come down.)

Scene Three

(Three weeks later. DANIELLE and SACHA are discovered standing, script in hand. THEY have just finished rehearsing a scene.)

SACHA: How did that feel? Any better?

DANIELLE: What do you think?

SACHA: I think when we lose the scripts you'll feel much more comfortable. You look tired. I think you should take some time off and relax. How about taking in a film tonight? Tell you what, I'll treat you to dinner? How's that?

DANIELLE: That's very kind of you.

SACHA: Nothing of the sort. I want you to be as happy as you can be, because the happier you are, the better you'll be, and the better you'll be, the better the production will be, and the better the production will be, the better I'll be, so I'm really a very selfish person. You don't believe me.

DANIELLE: No.

SACHA: You have a very suspicious nature.

DANIELLE: You must have done very well with the girls at Oxford.

SACHA: The French are not very popular in Great Britain.

DANIELLE: Oh, what a pity!

SACHA: You are heartless.

DANIELLE: Because I won't have dinner with you?

186

CHOICES

SACHA: This young man you're seeing, what is he like?

DANIELLE: Why do you want to know?

SACHA: I like to know what the competition is like.

DANIELLE: Surely you must have some lady friends here in Paris. You grew up here, didn't you?

SACHA: I've been away for two years.

DANIELLE: You've been back three weeks.

SACHA: People move. Some get married. Why are you so secretive about my competition? Is he as clever as I am?

DANIELLE: No.

SACHA: Is he as good looking as I am?

DANIELLE: No.

SACHA: Then what's the attraction?

DANIELLE: I make it a point not to get romantically involved with the people I'm working with.

SACHA: I don't see any engagement ring.

DANIELLE: He's very poor. He can't afford a ring.

SACHA: You're going to marry a pauper?

DANIELLE: He's a medical student.

SACHA: Oh, medical men are dreary. You'll be bored to tears

inside of a month. And it'll take years before he'll become a full fledged doctor.

DANIELLE: Haven't you ever been in love?

SACHA: I fell in love at the age of ten.

DANIELLE: *(Sarcastically)* At the age of ten? Really?

SACHA: I fell madly in love with this vision of pink and white. We were in the fourth grade, and every Saturday afternoon we'd go to the cinema together, and we'd hold hands. It was heaven.

DANIELLE: And what, pray tell, happened to this vision of pink and white?

SACHA: Her family moved away, and traitress that she was, she went right along with them.

DANIELLE: *(Sympathetically)* Ohhhhhh.

SACHA: And left me with a broken heart.

DANIELLE: Poor Sacha.

SACHA: It took me almost a year to get over it. As a matter of fact, I don't think I've ever gotten over it. It's left me very cynical about women.

DANIELLE: Then I think you ought to appreciate a woman who's as loyal as I am.

SACHA: Oh, but I do. That's what makes you so attractive.

DANIELLE: You are impossible.

CHOICES

SACHA: Won't you even have dinner with me, a poor lonely emigre?

DANIELLE: All right. I'll have dinner with you.

SACHA: This evening!

DANIELLE: On one condition.

SACHA: Uh, oh.

DANIELLE: You behave yourself, and don't make anymore of it than a friendly outing with a colleague.

(CLAUDETTE enters from the theatre.)

CLAUDETTE: Sacha, you're wanted for a fitting. Problem?

SACHA: No, no.

CLAUDETTE: Am I interrupting?

DANIELLE: No, no.

SACHA: She has all my costumes?

CLAUDETTE: There are only two. Marie is waiting.

SACHA: Rush, rush, rush. *(HE goes off.)*

CLAUDETTE: What's going on?

DANIELLE: He wants to take me to dinner.

CLAUDETTE: Have you told him?

189

CHOICES

DANIELLE: I told him I'm engaged.

CLAUDETTE: I'd leave it at that.

DANIELLE: Have you any suggestions, about my performance, I mean? Henri doesn't seem to be very pleased.

CLAUDETTE: Just take the time to find your way.

DANIELLE: Therese is rather heartless don't you think?

CLAUDETTE: She's intense, perhaps. And she loved her brother.

DANIELLE: But to kill someone, deliberately. She's different than I imagined her. I'm not sure that I'm the right actress for this role.

CLAUDETTE: Compassion, my dear.

DANIELLE: Compassion?

(HENRI enters from the theatre.)

HENRI: *(To CLAUDETTE)* Marie wants your opinion.

(CLAUDETTE goes off.)

HENRI: You look tired. Are we working you too hard?

DANIELLE: I haven't been sleeping too well.

HENRI: You'll be fine.

DANIELLE: I don't want to ruin your beautiful play.

HENRI: Don't worry about the play.

CHOICES

DANIELLE: If you want to replace me, I will understand. You've been so kind, and I feel that I'm not doing justice to the role.

HENRI: Let us be the judge of that.

DANIELLE: I've never played a murderess before.

HENRI: Is that how you see her?

DANIELLE: How do you see her, since you wrote her?

HENRI: There are some people to whom art is everything.

DANIELLE: More than life itself?

HENRI: Some people are willing to die for their country, to die for love.

DANIELLE: To die, yes. But to kill?

HENRI: A mother would kill to preserve the life of a child.

DANIELLE: I guess so.

HENRI: The publisher is a threat to the artistic life of his son because he refuses to support the boy so that the boy can write his novel.

DANIELLE: That's true.

HENRI: She also blames the publisher for the death of her brother. If the publisher had published her brother's novel, her brother would not have committed suicide.

DANIELLE: I see.

CHOICES

HENRI: And now she has the opportunity to preserve the artistic life of the publisher's son, who's in the same position her brother was.

(CLAUDETTE enters.)

CLAUDETTE: *(To DANIELLE)* Marie is ready for you now.

DANIELLE: What's that?

CLAUDETTE: Your costume.

DANIELLE: Oh. Yes, of course. Thank you. *(SHE goes off.)*

CLAUDETTE: Problem?

HENRI: She's a little confused.

CLAUDETTE: She's not the only one.

HENRI: What is that supposed to mean?

CLAUDETTE: Your mind seems to be elsewhere.

HENRI: If there's anyone who seems to be elsewhere, it's that son of yours. I'm very disappointed in Sacha. He's a frivolous child without a thought in that handsome head of his.

CLAUDETTE: When have I heard that before?

HENRI: I don't know. Maybe I was mistaken about Danielle, and Sacha could be in a comedy by Noel Coward. We should never have sent him to Oxford.

CLAUDETTE: Stop fretting. You're not even off book.

CHOICES

HENRI: And that's another thing.

CLAUDETTE: Then do me a favor. Concentrate on learning your lines. Let me look after the staging.

HENRI: It was a big mistake.

CLAUDETTE: What?

HENRI: The play. Sacha. Everything.

> *(HENRI goes off, into the living quarters. CLAUDETTE sighs, shakes her head and follows HENRI off as the lights come down.)*

ACT TWO

Scene One

(Monday evening. Two weeks later. SACHA, holding a script, enters from the theatre in costume and make-up. [The costumes are contemporary.] HE sits and checks speeches in the script. After a moment DANIELLE, holding a script, enters in costume and make-up. SHE sits, checks the script then lays it aside. There is a long silence. SACHA finally looks up at her.)

SACHA: Nervous?

DANIELLE: I'm petrified. You're as calm as a cucumber.

SACHA: Not really.

DANIELLE: Who's going to be out there?

SACHA: Friends.

DANIELLE: Theatre friends?

SACHA: Yes, of course.

DANIELLE: Like who?

SACHA: It all depends on who's in town.

DANIELLE: Like...?

SACHA: Jean Cocteau, Andre Gide, Mistinguett...

DANIELLE: That's enough.

SACHA: They're usually very supportive, really. And they'll love you.

194

CHOICES

DANIELLE: Therese is not very lovable.

SACHA: They'll love your performance.

DANIELLE: You think so?

SACHA: But then I'm prejudiced.

DANIELLE: You really are a wicked boy.

SACHA: Boy?

DANIELLE: Yes, boy.

SACHA: I suppose I am, from the vantage point of an old married woman.

DANIELLE: You haven't told your father, have you?

SACHA: I gave you my word.

DANIELLE: I've had some rather upsetting news. Ramon may be transferred...to another hospital.

SACHA: Will he be here tonight?

DANIELLE: He can only stay for the first act.

SACHA: Are your parents here?

DANIELLE: Oh, yes. and they're staying with us.

SACHA: In your little apartment?

DANIELLE: It's a nightmare. Poor Ramon. He has to sleep on the floor.

CHOICES

SACHA: Poor Ramon.

DANIELLE: Don't be mean. I'm really worried about him. He has to work so hard. He never gets any sleep. He's lost weight, and he looks so pale. I'll be so glad when his internship is over.

SACHA: You should have married an actor.

DANIELLE: Oh, yes. That would have really done the trick. Are you still seeing that little waitress?

SACHA: She's not a little waitress. She happens to be a budding Bernhardt.

DANIELLE: Oh, one of those.

SACHA: She's not the least bit phoney, if that's what you're getting at. As a matter of fact, she's really very sweet.

DANIELLE: I was only teasing. But you are very vulnerable.

SACHA: Yes, mother.

DANIELLE: My parents are all excited. Even my father's impressed, and he's usually very non-committal. "You're really appearing with Henri Prideaux?" *(After a moment.)* Do you think your father's pleased with my work? He never says very much.

SACHA: If he wasn't pleased, you'd hear about it.

DANIELLE: Sometimes he looks at me as if he's going to say something, then he looks away and says nothing.

SACHA: He's thinking.

DANIELLE: About what?

CHOICES

SACHA: About the set, the lights, the costumes, and about my performance.

DANIELLE: Isn't he pleased with your performance?

SACHA: He hasn't seen it yet, but he thinks he has, and he doesn't know what to do about it.

DANIELLE: I think you'll be fine, and you're certainly more secure than I am.

> (HENRI, holding a script, enters in costume. HE sits, glances at the script and lays it aside. HE looks at DANIELLE and smiles.)

HENRI: Ready?

DANIELLE: As ready as I'll ever be.

HENRI: Just remember, they are our guests. They've been invited.

DANIELLE: Yes! I know!

HENRI: The bigger they are, the nicer they are. *(After a moment.)* You're wearing a different blouse.

DANIELLE: The original blouse was green, and Marie said I couldn't wear it. She wouldn't tell me why.

HENRI: Ha!

DANIELLE: What?

HENRI: Moliere.

DANIELLE: Moliere?

CHOICES

HENRI: Moliere was performing in The Imaginary Invalid. He was deathly ill and barely finished the performance, and he died almost immediately afterwards.

SACHA: And the color of his costume was green.

HENRI: So it's considered safe to avoid wearing green. It's a ridiculous superstition, but why tempt fate?

(THEY sit in silence.)

DANIELLE: What time is it?

SACHA: Twenty five minutes to go.

DANIELLE: *(After a moment. To HENRI)* Bernhardt was your godmother, wasn't she?

HENRI: Oh, yes. and while she was alive there was a present at every birthday.

DANIELLE: Is it true that you attended the rehearsals for L'Aiglon?

HENRI: My father would take me along, and I would sit in a corner, open-mouthed.

DANIELLE: And Bernhardt really rehearsed a play for six months?

HENRI: Oh, yes.

DANIELLE: What took so long?

HENRI: Actually it was what you might call a social affair.

DANIELLE: For six months?

CHOICES

HENRI: The rehearsal was called for one. My father, who played Flambeau, would stroll in around two thirty. Rostand, the elegant playwright, would arrive half an hour later, and at ten to four Bernhardt made her entrance.

DANIELLE: What did they do in all that time?

HENRI: Sat around and told stories, just like we're doing now. And then when Madame arrived, the men would line up to kiss her hand. This took half an hour.

DANIELLE: To kiss her hand?

HENRI: There were sixty people in the cast.

DANIELLE: Goodness!

HENRI: And after that Bernhardt would retire to her dressing room to change into her costume...she always rehearsed in costume... and at five o'clock everything stopped. Madame Sarah had to have her tea. *(After a moment)* And oh yes! Once there was a great fuss about the horses.

DANIELLE: Horses?

HENRI: On the second day of rehearsal Bernhardt turned to Rostand. "What's this reference to a horse?" she asked. " It's a great distance," said Rostand. "You travel by horse." Not me," said Bernhardt. She was deathly afraid of horses. She finally agreed to try one; not to mount him, of course, just to lead him off. And when it turned out that there had to be two horses, one for her and one for my father, that was the end of the horses.

(THEY sit in silence.)

DANIELLE: What time is it?

CHOICES

SACHA: We still have ten minutes to go.

DANIELLE: Did you ever meet Rostand?

HENRI: Oh, yes. As a matter of fact, I heard Rostand himself, read the play, or most of it, at any rate.

DANIELLE: Oh?

HENRI: I was in the other room. I was about ten. They wanted my father for the role of Flambeau. Rostand himself came to read the play for Papa Maurice. Actually he didn't read the play, he performed it, and he gave an absolutely wonderful imitation of Sarah Bernhardt.

DANIELLE: Did he really?

HENRI: Oh, he was a wonderful actor. At any rate, when he finished the third act he stopped, exhausted...he was rather fragile, you know...and he looked up at my father. "Magnificent," said my father. "Well?" asked Rostand. "Well, yes," said my father, "I see no reason why I shouldn't appear in this wonderful play." And, of course, it really wasn't necessary for him to continue since the role of Flambeau never appeared again, which was why, we found out later, that Coquelin had turned it down.

(CLAUDETTE enters from the theatre holding a note pad.)

CLAUDETTE: Notes. *(SHE sits and consults the note pad.)* Henri, stop paraphrasing. It confuses the other actors.

HENRI: I apologize. I've had a lot on my mind.

CLAUDETTE: I'm aware of that, and so were you when you began to rehearse this play.

CHOICES

HENRI: Don't be cruel.

CLAUDETTE: "I mjust be cruel to be kind.", to quote the Master himself. Danielle, you must pick up your cues, especially in the opening scene. *(SHE consults her notes.)* Danielle...

DANIELLE: Yes?

CLAUDETTE: When you shoot Victor, don't hesitate. You know he's at the door. You've made up your mind. Shoot! In the opening of the second act you were late for your entrance.

DANIELLE: My shoe came off just before I entered.

CLAUDETTE: Is it too big?

DANIELLE: No, no. It's all right.

CLAUDETTE: Henri, in your final scene with David be decisive.

HENRI: I thought I was.

CLAUDETTE: That's all.

SACHA: No notes for me?

CLAUDETTE: No.

SACHA: You mean I'm perfect?

CLAUDETTE: Five minutes. Merde!

> *(SHE kisses the three of them on the cheek, SACHA then DANIELLE, then HENRI, then goes off.)*

SACHA: She's a tough lady.

CHOICES

HENRI: Why do you think I married her?

SACHA: So she could provide you with an heir.

HENRI: Think again. Group hug.

> (*HENRI rises and THEY form a circle, placing their arms about each others shoulders.*)

HENRI: (*To DANIELLE*) Shall we take our places.

> (*HENRI embraces SACHA emotionally and goes off. DANIELLE kisses SACHA on the cheek and follows HENRI off. SACHA sits up, alert. After a few moments, three knocks are heard offstage, the signal for the play to begin. The faint sound of thunder is heard.*)

HENRI: (*Very faintly, offstage*) Sorry about the weather.

> (*SACHA, deep in thought, leans forward, resting his elbows on his knees, as the lights come down.*)

(One o'clock the following afternoon. CLAUDETTE enters from the house, followed by HENRI. SHE carries a sheet of paper.)

HENRI: What's all the mystery?

CLAUDETTE: I'd like you to read this.

HENRI: What is it?

CLAUDETTE: A review.

HENRI: Of what?

CLAUDETTE: Kingdom By The Sea. I invited Andre Rochemont to the performance last night.

HENRI: Yes, my dear. I'm aware of that.

CLAUDETTE: You seemed so insecure...about the play, about everything, so I thought it wise to get an objective point of view.

HENR: An objective point of view? Andre Rochement?

CLAUDETTE: Henri, you know perfectly well, he's honest and intelligent. Are you going to read it or aren't you?

HENRI: No, I am not going to read it, and you should not have taken it upon yourself to invite that man.

CLAUDETTE: You're not going to read it?

HENRI: I am not going to read it.

CLAUDETTE: Then let me read it to you. I think you should hear what he has to say. Henri, you, yourself, weren't happy with what happened last night. Let me read it to you. Please.

HENRI: *(HE sits.)* Last night, I asked you how you thought it went, and you said, "Fine."

CLAUDETTE: What was I supposed to say with all our so-called friends standing around? Do you want to hear this, or shall I tear it up?

HENRI: Is he going to print it?

CLAUDETTE: Not necessarily

HENRI: What does that mean?

CLAUDETTE: He did it as a favor, for me.

HENRI: I see. And what did he get in return?

CLAUDETTE: You're not jealous, are you? Oh, really!

HENRI: Well, he has made a play for you, a number of times.

CLAUDETTE: I'm irresistible. Can I help it?

HENRI: You're an outrageous flirt. That's what you are. Oh, all right. Read the damn thing.

CLAUDETTE: He tried to be as objective...

HENRI: Without the prologue. If you don't mind, I would like to finish my lunch.

CLAUDETTE: *(SHE reads.)* "A Tragedy" That's the headline.

CHOICES

HENRI: Thank you.

CLAUDETTE: *(SHE continues to read.)* "Kingdom By The Sea, presented last night by Le Theatre Moderne, is a three character melodrama in which, by the final curtain, one character is still left standing. During this convoluted story a second character is murdered and, after committing the dastardly deed, the third character, the culprit, commits suicide.

HENRI: How perceptive!

CLAUDETTE: *(Continuing)* Actually, Danielle Moray, who portrays this hapless young murderess, is a lovely actress. Unfortunately she found herself in the wrong role, in the wrong play.

HENRI: Go on.

CLAUDETTE: *(Continuing)* She was not alone however. Since he was speaking words he should have been familiar with since he, himself, wrote the piece, the always dependable Henri Prideaux...

HENRI: Always dependable?

CLAUDETTE: *(Continuing)* The always dependable Henri Prideaux seemed slightly confused. I'm speaking now of Prideaux's performance, or rather the absence of one. We come now to this uncharacteristically gloomy melodrama from the pride and joy of boulevard comedy. This carefully crafted, joyless story, however...

HENRI: Carefully crafted?

CLAUDETTE: *(Continuing)* This carefully crafted, joyless story, however, centers on an intense young lady employed as an editor by a successful publisher. She kills her employer, so that his wastrel son will come into his father's wealth and be able to weather the shark infested waters of an artistic career. This, mind you. is partly in revenge for the suicide of the young lady's emotionally unstable brother who committed suicide because this same publisher turned down the beloved brother's novel. Oh yes, there's also an escaped lunatic in the area, a symbol, I assume, for something. I'm not quite sure what. There's also a good deal of thunder and lightning, darkness and candle light. As the curtain descends, the stage is filled with the rays of the rising sun to denote, I assume, that all's right with the world now that we've gotten rid of this awful mess.

HENRI: So articulate, so witty.

CLAUDETTE: *(Continuing)*...I've carefully omitted dealing with the third actor in this misbegotten production. The entire evening would have been a waste of time if not for the remarkably talented Sacha Prideaux.

HENRI: Aha!

CLAUDETTE: *(Continuing)* This young actor's performance as the publisher's son, was a revelation. But, perhaps, I should have expected this. Five years ago I attended a performance given by the students of the Academy Montfleur. It was a production of Hamlet with a sixteen year old Prideaux in the title role. The young man, the boy rather, gave an amazingly accomplished reading. It lacked, of course, a certain depth, but for one so young it was most impressive.

HENRI: What did I tell you?

CLAUDETTE: (Continuing)...So I must end up by saying that last night was, in one way, a theatrical event. We have witnessed the professional debut of a major star. In addition to a natural intelligence, young Prideaux has acquired an emotional depth so rare for a man of his age. This coupled with good looks, a

commanding presence and an ironic wit calls to mind the magic of
his grandfather, the great Maurice Prideaux. What would be most
exciting would be the return of young Prideaux in the role of
Hamlet, to which, I'll wager, he would bring a breath of fresh air.

HENRI: That's it?

CLAUDETTE: That's it.

HENRI: Now may I finish my lunch?

CLAUDETTE: You have nothing to say?

HENRI: It seems to me that your friend, the critic, has said it all.
What puzzles me is why you chose to invite a critic to a work in
progress. Especially a critic as caustic as Andre Rochemont.

CLAUDETTE: Since you yourself had misgivings, I thought it
wise to have an impartial view, before this production was exposed
to the light of day. I haven't shown this to anyone, and he's not
going to print it, unless you give him permission to.

HENRI: Thank you. And you can thank Andre as well.

CLAUDETTE: You can thank him yourself, since he wrote that
review as a personal favor.

(HENRI bursts out laughing.)

CLAUDETTE: You think that's funny?

HENRI: I laugh in order to hide my tears However I bow to your
perspicacity. I should have listened to you in the first place.

CLAUDETTE: Oh?

CHOICES

HENRI; You were right about Danielle. She's a lovely actress and, I must admit, I was a bit smitten. But she's really all wrong for Therese. I thought I could get a performance out of her. We both of us tried, but it was a fatal mistake and, as a result of this crucial piece of miscasting, and my slipshod performance, the play doesn't work.

CLAUDETTE: Are you going to replace her?

HENRI: At the moment I'm going to finish my lunch. May I have that review?

CLAUDETTE: Yes, of course.

HENRI: Thank you.

> (*CLAUDETTE hands the review to HENRI who folds it, places it in his coat pocket and goes off to the living quarters. DANIELLE enters from the theatre.*)

DANIELLE: I'm sorry I'm late.

CLAUDETTE: That's quite all right. We won't be starting on time.

DANIELLE: I'm glad I caught you alone. I have some rather upsetting news. Ramon is being transferred to a hospital in Bordeaux, and I don't know what to do.

CLAUDETTE: Have you had your lunch?

DANIELLE: No. I was too upset. He leaves tomorrow and I was helping him pack. They're giving him his own apartment, and he wants me to come with him.

CLAUDETTE: One never knows, my dear. Sometimes these things work out for the best.

CHOICES

DANIELLE: How can you say that? Last night was so exciting, so wonderful, meeting all those distinguished people. And, to top it all off, Andre Rochement was there, and he loved my performance, and he flirted with me outrageously.

CLAUDETTE: Yes, well, that's Andre for you.

DANIELLE: Ramon has no choice, it's true, but then, for that matter, neither do I. I've made a commitment. And my parents simply don't understand. *(Tearfully)* They insist my place is with Ramon. But it's not as if he'll be living in another country. There are trains, there are busses, there are telephones. And besides, he'll be busy and so will I. As a matter of fact, this may be the perfect test. If what we feel for one another is so fragile, then the sooner we find out the better. What do you think? Tell me truthfully.

CLAUDETTE: I have made it a hard and fast rule, when it comes to affairs of the heart, never give advice to anyone. I suggest you have something to eat first, and then, who knows, it may all work out for the best.

DANIELLE: You're right, of course. But why does life have to be so complicated?

(SACHA enters from the living quarters.)

SACHA: Good morning.

(DANIELLE marches off.)

SACHA: What was that all about?

CLAUDETTE: Personal problems.

SACHA: Aha!

CHOICES

CLAUDETTE: What is that supposed to mean?

(SACHA shrugs.)

CLAUDETTE: She confided in you?

SACHA: Then you know?

CLAUDETTE: Yes, of course.

SACHA: And?

CLAUDETTE: He's being transferred to a hospital in Bordeaux.

SACHA: Oh, poor Danielle! Incidentally, what was Andre Rochemont doing here last night? You didn't invite him, did you?

CLAUDETTE: Yes.

SACHA: Since when did you start inviting critics to a private performance?

CLAUDETTE: I thought we needed an objective eye.

SACHA: He's not going to write a review, is he?

CLAUDETTE: He's written one.

SACHA: Oh? Where is it?

CLAUDETTE: Your father has it.

SACHA: Aha! And from the look on Papa's face, it couldn't be very good.

CLAUDETTE: That should please you.

CHOICES

SACHA: Now why would you say a thing like that?

CLAUDETTE: You're a selfish child, and it's probably my fault.

SACHA: I had a long talk with Rochemont last night. Or, rather, he had a long talk with me. He thought my performance was a breath of fresh air.

CLAUDETTE: That must have pleased you.

SACHA: He thinks I'm needed here.

CLAUDETTE: And what did you say?

SACHA: I agreed.

CLAUDETTE: I see.

SACHA: But then I said that I didn't think there was room for me here.

CLAUDETTE: Oh? Is that what you said?

SACHA: Mama, this theatre happens to be a one man operation. Henri Prideaux **is** The Theatre Moderne. He writes, he produces, he directs and he is its star. There's no room for anyone else.

CLAUDETTE: As the years go by, my dear, we human stars, unlike the stars in the heavens, begin to wane. You are needed here.

(DANIELLE enters accompanied by HENRI.)

HENRI: So, here we are. Sit down. The response to Kingdom By the Sea was not what I had hoped for. But then, that's what we need an audience for. I still think that Kingdom By The Sea may be the best play I've written. However, I'm going to lay it aside, for the moment. Which means, of course, that you, Danielle, are released.

DANIELLE: Oh?

HENRI: You'll be receiving a check for the additional four weeks.

DANIELLE: Thank you.

HENRI: You're a very talented young actress, and I'm sure you'll go far, and I'll be happy to write you a letter of reference.

DANIELLE: Does this mean there are no additional performances of Kingdom By The Sea?

HENRI: For the present. You are free.

DANIELLE: I see.

HENRI: Don't look so sad, my dear. I see a great future for you.

DANIELLE: Then, if you don't mind, I'd like to leave. I have some things to attend to.

HENRI: Yes, of course. I've arranged for a farewell dinner tomorrow evening for the entire company. We'll be dining at Maxim's. Feel free to bring a friend.

DANIELLE: That's very kind of you, but my friend is leaving town tomorrow and, the way it looks now, since there's nothing to keep me here, I'll be joining him.

HENRI: Oh?

CHOICES

DANIELLE: He's a medical student and he's being transferred to a hospital in Bordeaux.

HENRI: I see.

DANIELLE: *(SHE looks at the three of them.)* I'm going to miss you.

SACHA: We'll miss you, too.

HENRI: Now, now, now. No tears.

(SHE embraces HENRI, then SACHA and CLAUDETTE.)

CLAUDETTE: You will write to us, won't you?

DANIELLE: Yes, of course. Oh, God! I'll miss you so, all of you. *(SHE runs off.)*

SACHA: Poor Danielle. I hope she's happy there.

HENRI: Why shouldn't she be? If she's following him to Bordeaux, she must be in love with the boy.

SACHA: Would you be happy in Bordeaux?

HENRI: I've played Bordeaux. It's not the end of the world.

CLAUDETTE: And she will be with her husband.

HENRI: She's married? Amazing. It just goes to show. You think you know someone, and you don't know them at all. She's married, and you knew it?

(CLAUDETTE nods.)

CHOICES

HENRI: Why did she keep it such a secret?

CLAUDETTE: You made such a fuss about Dora being pregnant.

SACHA: She was so excited about this production. This was her big break.

CLAUDETTE: I think she's lucky.

HENRI: Why?

CLAUDETTE: She was about to make a decision which might have led, I think, to a very difficult situation.

HENRI: Love and art. Civilians don't understand, do they? Now that's an idea for a play. Love and art, the choices we make. At any rate, here we are! The opening two weeks away, and we have no play. Of course, we could always revive A Private Affair.

CLAUDETTE: Oh, really!

HENRI: What?

CLAUDETTE: Don't you think we're a little long in the tooth for those roles?

HENRI: Nonsense. Lucy and Ronald could be any age. They are ageless.

CLAUDETTE: Unfortunately, we aren't Lucy and Ronald, two characters in a play. We are human beings, of a definite age which, incidentally, the public is well aware of. What about Andre's suggestion?

HENRI: What suggestion is that? Oh.

CHOICES

SACHA: What was Andre's suggestion?

HENRI: Hamlet.

SACHA: What a great idea!

HENRI: Why do you think I left the Comedie Francaise? One classic after another. Moliere, Corneille, Racine. A theatre should present new plays, exciting work that's never been seen before.

SACHA: Over the past ten years the public has seen a lot of new plays, a lot of, primarily, Henri Prideaux.

CLAUDETTE: Sacha!

HENRI: That's all right. He's right. As a matter of fact, at this point, I suppose, presenting a classic might actually be a refreshing change.

SACHA: It would take me a week or two to brush up on Hamlet. And you'd make a wonderful Claudius, or even Polonius.

HENRI: Polonius?!

SACHA: And Mama would make a lovely Gertrude.

CLAUDETTE: I'd love to play Gertrude. And, I agree with Sacha. You'd make a wonderful Claudius.

HENRI: But Hamlet.

SACHA: *(To CLAUDETTE)* I told you.

HENRI: What?

CHOICES

SACHA: Papa, do you or do you not want me to join the company?

HENRI: But Hamlet.

SACHA: It's no use. I told you.

CLAUDETTE: Henri, sit down and listen to the boy.

SACHA: I am not a boy, and I would love to join the company, but it would have to be as a partner, an equal partner. And I would insist on performing all the great roles, like Hamlet, Cyrano, Alceste in The Misanthrope.

HENRI: Hamlet, Cyrano and The Misanthrope?

SACHA: Among others.

HENRI: All in one season?

SACHA: Not necessarily. However, if you want me in the company, you would have to agree to my terms.

CLAUDETTE: Last season, my dear, was not a huge success. With Sacha performing the great roles in the classics we might attract a new audience, and audience that we haven't reached before.

HENRI: Let me think about it.

SACHA: I agreed to come back for Kingdom By The Sea because you said you'd written the role for me, and Mama insisted so here I am. However, now that Kingdom By The Sea is no more, I feel free to return to Great Britain...unless...

HENRI: Unless we do Hamlet.

CHOICES

SACHA: Not only Hamlet. I must be free to choose at least one play a season.

HENRI: I see. Apparently you've given the matter a great deal of thought. And is there room for an old veteran in these plans of yours?

SACHA: Yes, of course. A talented actor and a playwright as well. What more could a company ask for?

HENRI: Thank you.

SACHA: I suggest we draw up a contract.

HENRI: A contract?

SACHA: Between the two of us, a contract that we both can live with.

CLAUDETTE: I think that's an excellent idea.

HENRI: A contract, between a father and a son?

SACHA: Between two business partners.

HENRI: Let me think about it.

SACHA: I've still got that copy of Hamlet with all my notes. *(HE goes off.)*

HENRI: That boy of yours is...

CLAUDETTE: What?

HENRI: Rather frightening.

CHOICES

CLAUDETTE: And you were right all along. You said that as soon as he got back up on that stage he'd be hooked.

HENRI: Did I say that? Ah well.

CLAUDETTE: Ah well, what?

HENRI: Be careful what you wish for.

CLAUDETTE: Oh, stop it! You're delighted, and you know it. Andre's waiting for my call. I'll tell him not to print the review.

HENRI: Don't be ridiculous. What better publicity for our production of Hamlet?! And you might add that in the Spring, by which time, I will know mky lines, I'll be producing a revised version of Kingdom By The Sea, with Dora in the role of Therese. In addition to that there's going to be a new comedy starring Henri Prideaux and Claudette Duval.

CLAUDETTE: Oh? What's it to be about?

HENRI: I'm not quite sure. Love and art, perhaps, the choices one makes. Or...

CLAUDETTE: Or what?

HENRI: The attempt of a critic to seduce a famous actress who's married to a famous playwright who's jealous of the critic.

CLAUDETTE: Thank God!

HENRI: For what?.

CLAUDETTE: That you're still jealous.

CHOICES

(CLAUDETTE kisses HENRI and goes off. HENRI sits lost in thought as the lights come down.)

THE PROPER TECHNIQUE
A Romantic Comedy

CAST OF CHARACTERS

May Strauss

Jack Gardner

George Butterfield

Leo Strauss

Jenny Strauss

SCENE

Living room of Jack Gardner's apartment in New York City

TIME

A few decades ago

ACT ONE

Scene One

(The living room of JACK GARDNER's apartment on Central Park West in Manhattan. It is a luxurious, tastefully furnished room. A door stage right leads to the rest of the apartment. A door upstage center leads to the outside corridor. French doors stage left leads to a terrace. There are a couple of original impressionist paintings on the wall. The decor is elegant and simple.
It is early afternoon of a pleasant day in May. The doorbell rings. GEORGE BUTTERFIELD, a tall, sharp-featured man, rather esthetic looking, mid thirties, enters from the terrace. HE is in his shirtsleeves, wears a dark, heavy apron and carries a watering can. HE opens the outer door and MAY STRAUSS, a delightful child of nineteen, is discovered in the doorway. HE eyes her suspiciously.)

MAY: You're...George Butterfield.

GEORGE: So I've been told.

MAY: Do you live here?

GEORGE: No, I work here. I'm Mr. Gardner's private secretary.

MAY: But you're a fine actor. Why would you be working as a secretary?

GEORGE: That's what I keep asking myself. Unfortunately actors do have to eat.

MAY: That's disgraceful. Why doesn't Mr. Gardner use you in his pictures?

222

THE PROPER TECHNIQUE

GEORGE: He does, whenever he can. And who, may I ask, are you?

MAY: I'm May. May...Starling. I'm here to interview Mr. Gardner. If you're his secretary, you should be aware of that.

GEORGE: You're a little early, aren't you?

MAY: I'm always early. It's a terrible habit. But I think being late is worse. Don't you? I'm with the Herald.

GEORGE: Tribune?

MAY: No. The Columbia Herald. I'm a student at Columbia University.

GEORGE: And you're on the Herald.

MAY: Can you keep a secret? I'm not really on the Herald, but I thought they really should have an article about Mr. Gardner since, it looks like he's going to spend some time here in New York. You won't give me away, will you?

GEORGE: I really should.

MAY: After the nice things I said about you?

GEORGE: How old are you?

MAY: You never ask a lady her age.

GEORGE: You look like you ought to be in grammar school.

MAY: Oh, I know. It's a curse. But it's the face I was born with, so what can I do? Are we going to stand here in the doorway?

GEORGE: Oh, I'm sorry.

MAY: That's quite all right.

(SHE enters the room and looks about. HE closes the door.)

GEORGE: I hope you approve.

MAY: It must be nice to be that rich.

GEORGE: It's better than being poor.

MAY: Is that an original Modigliani?

GEORGE: I hope so.

(JACK GARDNER, a handsome man in his thirties, enters from the interior, wearing a sports shirt and slacks.)

JACK: George...? Oh, I beg your pardon. Who have we here?

GEORGE: This is your two o'clock appointment.

JACK: Miss...?

MAY: Starling.

JACK: You're the reporter?

MAY: I'm afraid so.

THE PROPER TECHNIQUE

JACK: From the Herald?

GEORGE: The Columbia Herald. She's a student at the university.

JACK: Oh, I see.

GEORGE: Don't look at me. You were the one who made the appointment.

JACK: Did I?

GEORGE: Benny Segal.

JACK: Oh, yes. You're a friend of Benny's?

MAY: He's a friend of the family.

JACK: Well, any friend of Benny's is a friend of mine.

GEORGE: Well, I'll leave you two friends...to conduct your business.

JACK: Where did you get that ridiculous apron?

GEORGE: I bought it. That is, I bought it, and you paid for it. The last time I watered your plants I wet myself.

JACK: We can't have that, now can we?

GEORGE: And now, if you'll excuse me, I do have a life of my own. I've answered the mail. I've watered the plants, and now I would like to take in the sights.

THE PROPER TECHNIQUE

JACK: You're not going to wander about in that apron all day. Give it here.

GEORGE: *(HE hands the apron to JACK, and turns to MAY.)* Do I need a jacket?

MAY: Oh, no. It's a beautiufl day.

GEORGE: Good luck. *(HE goes off.)*

MAY: You really should make more use of him... I mean in your pictures.

JACK: You think so?

MAY: Don't you think he's talented?

JACK: I've thought so for years. We were students together.

MAY: Ah, the theatre, the theatre! It's so precarious.

JACK: You're not really a reporter, are you?

MAY: I don't pretend to be.

JACK: Then why are you here, may I ask?

MAY: Well, I just thought that....

JACK: I've upset you. I'm sorry.

MAY: Do you know how much courage it took me to come up here? I mean, after all, you are Jack Gardner, and I'm...

THE PROPER TECHNIQUE

JACK: A friend of Benny Segal's.

(THEY laugh.)

JACK: I'm sorry. I didn't mean to frighten you. Am I that imposing?

MAY: Since I've only seen you on the screen, and you're very big up there.

JACK: I sometimes forget. Now, young lady, do you have a list of questions you'd like to ask me?

MAY: What's that? Oh, yes. *(SHE fumbles in her purse, pulling out several things and finally coming up with a note pad.)*

JACK: Would you care for drink? I have some ginger ale, and there may be a coke.

MAY: A glass of wine might be nice.

JACK: How old are you?

MAY: I'm nineteen.

JACK: I don't believe it.

MAY: I can show you my drivers license.

JACK: Okay.

(SHE produces a driver's license and shows it to him.)

JACK: You've got your thumb over your name.

THE PROPER TECHNIQUE

MAY: *(Her thumb firmly in place)* Is that my picture, or is it not? And you can see my age.

JACK: Okay, okay. But you do look like a child.

MAY: I know what I look like, but I assure you, I'm not.

JACK: What would you like? To drink?

MAY: You wouldn't, by any chance, have Moltepuciano?

JACK: Moltepuciano?

MAY: Never mind. A merlot or a cabernet will do.

> *(HE goes to the liquor cabinet, pours her a glass of wine and hands it to her.)*

MAY: Thank you. Aren't you going to join me?

JACK: Yes. Yes, of course. *(HE pours himself some wine.)* To your success...with the Herald.

MAY: Thank you.

> *(THEY drink.)*

JACK: Well, shall we start?

> *(MAY sets her glass down.)*

JACK: You're trembling. Are you all right?

MAY: Yes. Yes, I'm fine. It's just that I've suddenly realized that

THE PROPER TECHNIQUE

I'm sitting here with Jack Gardner, and actually carrying on a conversation with him. I'm being silly, I know, because, after all, you are just an ordinary human being. I mean, after all, you are... just another actor.

JACK: Well...

MAY: With faults, just like anyone else. What I mean to say is, you have been married twice. Not that I'm standing in judgement.

JACK: Thank you.

MAY: And maybe it wasn't your fault. The divorces, I mean.

JACK: Thank you.

MAY: I mean a man in your position...and I'm sure you have your weaknesses, just like everyone else. Of course, you've got to take part of the blame, though fame does do things to people.

JACK: You think so?

MAY: I know so.

JACK: You're very wise for your age. What are you smiling at?

MAY: I can see you saying that in one of your movies, with just that same expression. "The Divorce" with Irene Dunne. *(Imitating him)* "You're very wise for your age." Or the one with Myrna Loy.

JACK: Have you seen all of my movies?

MAY: At least twice.

THE PROPER TECHNIQUE

JACK: You're a fan.

MAY: Well, of course, I am. Why do you think I'm here? I mean, why do you think I chose you for my interview?

JACK: Have you ever interviewed anyone before? Are you feeling all right?

MAY: *(SHE puts her hand to her mouth.)* Would you excuse me? *(SHE looks about.)*

JACK: It's right through there, to the left.

> *(MAY goes off quickly. JACK picks up the phone and dials.)*

GEORGE: Can I speak to Benny, please? It's Jack Gardner. *(After a moment)* Benny, what are you trying to do to me? Who is this child you sent me? Oh? Well, why didn't you say so? I see. No, no, no. Everything's fine, just fine. Listen, you haven't leaked anything about my doing a play, have you? I'm just asking. Okay, okay. As a matter of fact, I was thinking of getting in touch with Leo Strauss. Right. Right. I've got to go.

> *(JACK hangs up as MAY reenters.)*

JACK: Everything okay?

MAY: I'm fine. I'm sorry I made such a fool of myself.

JACK: Are you really a student at Columbia?

MAY: I'm a junior. I'm sorry. I'm much too nervous to be able to conduct an interview, much less write one. It took all my courage to get this far, and I'm afraid I've run out of steam. I won't take up anymore of your time.

JACK: Where are you rushing off to?

MAY: You must have more important things to attend to.

JACK: As a matter of fact, I have nothing to attend to. And I'd be happy if you could join me for lunch.

MAY: Lunch? It's almost two thirty.

JACK: Have you had your lunch?

MAY: That was my lunch that I left in your bathroom.

JACK: Then you must be hungry. I can't let you leave with an empty stomach, now can I. Why don't you join me, for a light snack.

MAY: Would you like me to?

JACK: It's settled then. What would you like? A salad, perhaps. That's what I'm going to have. A cobb salad and iced tea. How does that sound?

MAY: A small salad maybe?

JACK: A small salad it is. (HE picks up the phone and dials.)
Mr. Gardner, Henry. Would you send up two cobb salads. Make one a small one. And two iced teas. Thank you. (HE hangs up.)
Now, tell me about yourself. What are you studying?

MAY: Do you really want to know?

THE PROPER TECHNIQUE

JACK: Not if you don't want to talk about it.

MAY: Why don't we talk about you?

JACK: What would you like to know?

MAY: Why don't we begin at the beginning?

JACK: You'll have to be more specific.

MAY: Your family.

JACK: I have one brother and one sister, both happily married and well grounded. I have two nephews and one niece.

MAY: Are your parents alive?

JACK: Oh, yes.

MAY: Are they happily married too?

JACK: When I say happily married, I mean that a couple is still together. I'm not quite sure there is such a thing as a happy marriage. I take that back. A truly happy marriage is very, very rare.

MAY: You're speaking from experience, of course.

JACK: Experience and observation.

MAY: Do you think you'll ever marry again?

JACK: Probably.

THE PROPER TECHNIQUE

MAY: Why, if you're first two experiences were a disaster? Or is that too strong a word?

JACK: If I'm going to get the third degree, I've got to fortify myself. *(HE takes a sip of his wine.)* Would you like something else?

MAY: No, thank you. Why would you marry again, if you have such a jaundiced opinion of marriage.

JACK: Because the first year of my first marriage was the happiest year of my life.

MAY: You were in love with her, your first wife?

JACK: Oh, yes.

MAY: What happened?

JACK: We met in an ivory tower, the campus of Ohio State University, and then there was the cruel world, the agonizing, uncertainty of life as an actor. Nancy was a little too fragile for that, I'm afraid.

MAY: You're still in love with her, aren't you?

JACK: I guess I always will be.

MAY: Is there any chance...?

JACK: No, no, no. She's since remarried and has three healthy children. Or so I've been told. I've never met them, nor have I met her husband.

THE PROPER TECHNIQUE

MAY: The parting was a bitter one.

JACK: For me it was. Not that I blame her. Don't look so sad. It's not the end of the world.

MAY: Apparently, for you, it wasn't.

JACK: Yes, well, Arlene was a mistake. I married her on the rebound. She's an actress, you know. At least she claims to be.

MAY: Actors are children, aren't they?

JACK: What do you know about actors?

MAY: I haven't been completely honest with you. And I swore Uncle Benny to secrecy, but Leo Strauss is my father.

JACK: Is he really?

(The doorbell rings.)

JACK: That must be our lunch. Excuse me. *(HE opens the door, stands in the doorway, receives a large tray, mutters "Thank you." and closes the door. HE places the tray on the coffee table, brings over a small table then places the tray on the table, then places two chairs around the table.)* Shall we?

(THEY sit at the table.)

MAY: I'm really not very hungry.

JACK: Then you can just pick. Isn't that from some play or other. "I'll just pick."

THE PROPER TECHNIQUE

MAY: You were talking about your second wife.

JACK: That's enough about me. As the daughter of Leo Strauss I'm sure your life must be very...colorful.

MAY: It is that.

JACK: What was that sigh all about?

MAY: Life at home can be very exhausting. Between Daddy and Jenny. That's my mother. She doesn't like to be referred to as Mother. I guess you might say we're Bohemians.

JACK: And you've never been bitten...by the acting bug, I mean?

MAY: For one very brief moment, when I was little. And I decided then and there that the stage was not for me. I'm a great disappointment to Jenny. But I feel that there's got to be one sane one in the family.

JACK: And what about your father?

MAY: Daddy lives in another world. And I'm just one of his many children. I'm speaking figuratively, of course.

JACK: You feel neglected.

MAY: Oh, no. I'm greatly relieved. I prefer to watch the circus.

JACK: Your father's quite an important man.

MAY: Yes, I know. You've never met him?

JACK: No. No I haven't. I did hear him speak once, and I was very impressed.

MAY: Daddy's very dedicated.

JACK: And as a father?

MAY: He's very dedicated.

JACK: And...Jenny?

MAY: A force of nature. Which reminds me. I'd better call her. May I use your phone?

JACK: Yes, of course.

(MAY picks up the phone and dials.)

MAY: Hello? Nora? Is Jenny there? Thank you? Yes, Jenny, I'm fine. I'm having lunch with Jack Gardner. Why should I lie? Jenny, I am not making this up. Would you like to speak to him? All right. Hold on. *(SHE turns to JACK.)* She thinks I'm imagining things. Would you mind speaking to her? *(SHE hands the phone to JACK.)*

JACK: Hello? Yes, I'm afraid it is. No, no. Your daughter is absolutely charming. She's here to interview me for her university paper. No, no, no. She's no trouble at all. As a matter of fact, we're getting along splendidly. Thank you. No, no. I'm in town to stay...for quite some time. This evening? That's very kind of you, but what about tomorrow evening? Or if you'd care to stop by for an after dinner drink this evening. I'm expecting some calls from the coast early on. I have an apartment at the Whitaker. Any time that's convenient. I'll be in all evening. That'll be fine. No, I've never met Mr. Strauss, but I'm a great admirer of his work. I look forward to it. Would you like to speak to May? Hold on. *(HE hands the phone to MAY.)*

MAY: Yes, Jenny. Yes, I'm listening. I'll be home for dinner. I've got to stop at the library, and then I'll come home. We'll talk then. *(SHE sighs, closes her eyes and listens.)* Right. Right. I'll see you later. *(SHE hangs up.)*

JACK: What was that all about?

MAY: You don't want to know.

JACK: Mothers sometimes can be a problem.

MAY: Jenny is not just a mother. Jenny is THE mother of all mothers.

JACK: What is your father like...at home, I mean?

MAY: Absent-minded.

JACK: You haven't touched your salad.

MAY: I'm much too excited to eat. I really should be going.

JACK: Will you come by this evening, with your parents?

MAY: Would you like me to?

JACK: Yes, I would.

MAY: I do have some studying to do.

THE PROPER TECHNIQUE

JACK: Tell you what? I'll try to dig up a bottle of... What was that again?

MAY: Moltepuciano.

JACK: Moltepuciano.

MAY: In that case...I'll try. Thank you for being so patient with me.

JACK: It's been my pleasure.

MAY: I'm sure it has.

JACK: No, no. I mean it. You're a charming young lady.

MAY: *(SHE smiles.)* Okay.

JACK: It's been a pleasure.

MAY: You said that.

JACK: Only because you seem to need reassurance.

(HE sees her to the door and opens it.)

MAY: Enjoy your cobb salad. *(SHE goes off.)*

JACK: Thank you.

(JACK closes the door then sits down and starts on the salad. HE stops, rises, goes to the phonograph and puts on a record. We hear a romantic ballad. HE goes back to the table, sits thoughtfully and listens to the music, then sits up

238

and attacks his salad as the lights come down. The music continues throughout the scene change.)

Scene Two

(Nine o'clock that evening. The room is empty. GEORGE enters from the outside carrying a plastic bag.)

JACK: *(Offstage)* George?

GEORGE: Who else could it be?.

JACK: *(Offstage)* Did you have any trouble?

GEORGE: None whatsoever. *(HE removes two bottles of wine from the bag and places them on the bar.)*

JACK: *(Offstage)* You sure you got the right one?

GEORGE: Moltepuciano. Whoever heard of Moltepuciano?

(JACK enters from the interior.)

JACK: May. *(HE inspects the bottle.)*

GEORGE: Don't you trust me?

JACK: I was just curious. Moltepuciano. Abruzzo.

GEORGE: Let me ask you something. As a matter of fact, I'm afraid to ask. You don't, by any chance, have designs on that little snippet?

JACK: Don't be ridiculous. She's half my age.

GEORGE: I'm glad you're aware of that. What?

JACK: Nothing.

THE PROPER TECHNIQUE

GEORGE: What time are you expecting them?

JACK: Nine thirty or so.

GEORGE: Is she coming too?

JACK: By she, I suppose you mean May. Possibly.

GEORGE: Possibly?

JACK: Possibly. She has homework to do. She is a student, you know.

GEORGE: I am very well aware of that. I am also aware of the fact that you need a nursemaid. You know, sometimes I think you don't really know the difference between real life and the roles you play.

JACK: I'm a romantic. Can I help it? I'm very nervous.

GEORGE: He is not a god, you know.

JACK: In some circles, he is.

GEORGE: You're not thinking of studying with him.

JACK: I'm sure he's much too busy to take on anyone else.

GEORGE: Don't say I didn't warn you. Do you want me to stick around?

JACK: Not if you don't want to.

(The doorbell rings. GEORGE looks at his watch.)

THE PROPER TECHNIQUE

GEORGE: They're early. Do you want me to answer the door?

(GEORGE hesitates, then opens the door. JENNY STRAUSS, a full-bodied, exotic looking woman in her late forties, is discovered. Barely discernible behind her is LEO STRAUSS, a fastidious man with rather delicate features, in his early fifties.)

GEORGE: Greetings. I'm Mr. Gardner's assistant.

JENNY: You're George Butterfield.

GEORGE: That, too. Won't you come in?

(JENNY, followed by LEO, enters and approaches JACK. SHE sighs and extends her hands.)

JENNY: You really look like that.

JACK: I'm afraid so.

JENNY: Even better, I think. *(SHE glances from GEORGE to JACK)* Are you two...?

GEORGE: What?

JENNY: Never mind. It's a lovely apartment. How many rooms do you have?

JACK: Seven.

JENNY: My favorite Modigliani. That's the original?

JACK: Yes, it is. How do you do?

THE PROPER TECHNIQUE

(JACK extends his hand. JENNY kisses him on both cheeks.)

JENNY: In New York, we kiss.

(JACK extends his hand to LEO. LEO shakes it.)

LEO: Some of us just shake hands.

JACK: It's so nice of you to come. I'm very flattered.

JENNY: I must warn you. We're not the high falutin' type, like your Hollywood crowd.

LEO: My wife does her best to shock people.

JENNY: I say what I think.

LEO: If only you thought before you said it.

JENNY: We're a comedy team. Or so we've been told. So? You're turning your back on la la land?

JACK: Not quite.

JENNY: You're not gonna do a show?

LEO: Jenny!

JENNY: What? I'm just asking. If you don't ask, how will you know? Why are we standing? Are we allowed to sit?

JACK: Please.

THE PROPER TECHNIQUE

(JENNY and LEO sit.)

JENNY: So why are you in New York if you're not gonna do a show?

LEO: Jenny!

JENNY: Leo, please. I know what I'm doing.

JACK: As a matter of fact...

JENNY: I knew it. What did I tell you? Eventually they all come to their senses. Those with intelligence and talent, that is.

JACK: Am I included in that category?

JENNY: You're at the top. As everyone, who knows anything, knows that comedy is the hardest. Tragedy you just let it all out. Comedy needs a little thought, and the proper technique.

JACK: And what might that be?

JENNY: Leo, tell him.

LEO: I don't think Mr. Gardner needs me to tell him anything about the technique of comedy.

JENNY: You have a terrace. Oh, let me look.

(GEORGE escorts JENNY to the terrace and opens the French doors.)

JENNY: Oh, my God, what a view! Leo, come look. It's like magic. Did you ever see anything so beautiful. And what a night!

THE PROPER TECHNIQUE

(JENNY steps out onto the terrace, followed by GEORGE.)

LEO: You must excuse my wife. She really has a heart of gold. The trouble is...sometimes it glitters too brightly.

JACK: It's a great honor to meet you, sir.

LEO: Please. We are colleagues, men of the theatre. I include film work as theatre nowadays. We used to look down on Hollywood in the early days. Now more than half of us are out there, toiling in Babylon.

JACK: I've heard so much about you. I must admit, I'm a little in awe. The fact is I am thinking about doing a play.

LEO: An original?

JACK: I don't have that much courage. No, I've always been fond of The Affairs Of Anatol.

LEO: Schnitzler. A favorite of mine.

JACK: Do you know The Affairs Of Anatol?

LEO: But of course. A very wise choice. Also an opportunity to enlist the aid of some lovely young ladies.

JACK: So you really think that would be a good choice.

LEO: Offhand, I can't think of a better one. There's something poignant about a fickle man who longs for commitment.

JACK: You think he's a fickle man?

THE PROPER TECHNIQUE

LEO: He's a man. Aren't all men fickle? Not that all of us have the courage to act on our baser instincts, or can afford to...as Anatol could. The Affairs of Anatol, of course, is a social commentary.

JACK: That never occurred to me.

LEO: There's no reason why it should. As an actor you have enough to deal with.

JACK: You think it's a difficult role?

LEO: If acting were easy, my friend, we would all be Laurence Oliviers. Not that Larry's technique quite meshes with the reality of his role. And not that his method is one that I approve of.

JACK: And what might that be?

LEO: Approaching a role from the outside in.

JACK: Instead of from the inside out.

LEO: Exactly. But you've been on the stage. And if you're planning to come to Broadway I'm sure you know what you're doing.

JACK: That's just it. I haven't been on a stage for over eight years.

LEO: It'll come back to you.

JACK: You think so?

(JENNY reenters, followed by GEORGE.)

JACK: Would anyone care for a drink? I've just discovered a new wine. Moltepuciano.

THE PROPER TECHNIQUE

JENNY: You, too?

LEO: What do you mean, "you too"?

JENNY: Your daughter. She suddenly prides herself on being continental.

LEO: I understand you met our daughter this afternoon. I hope she wasn't a pest. She's a great fan of yours.

JACK: No, no, no. May is...a charming girl.

LEO: We think so. Even though she's a great disappointment.

JENNY: He wanted a boy.

LEO: Thank you, Mr. Winchell. No, the fact of the matter is my daughter has no real interest in the theatre.

JENNY: You mean she doesn't want to be an actress. As if there aren't enough actresses in the world...your world especially. The fact is, May is a wonderful actress in real life, just as I am. Acting need not be confined to the stage. Isn't that so, George?

GEORGE: Why, yes. I suppose so.

JENNY: You didn't hear a word I said.

LEO: Then he must be deaf.

GEORGE: Why don't I do the honors? Mr. Strauss, what would you care to drink?

LEO: Scotch on the rocks, if that's available.

THE PROPER TECHNIQUE

GEORGE: *(HE starts to prepare the drink.)* Jenny?

JENNY: Do you have any brandy...or a liqueur?

GEORGE: We've got Cointreau and Grand Marnier.

JENNY: Grand Marnier.

GEORGE: Ice?

JENNY: Never.

> *(GEORGE serves LEO his drink, then pours the Grand Marnier.)*

JACK: I know you've had your dinner, but I do have some nuts and some fruit. *(HE goes off.)*

JENNY: How long have you been working for Jack?

GEORGE: About a year or so. Ever since his divorce.

JENNY: The first or the second?

LEO: He said a year or so.

JENNY: You've never been married?

GEORGE: Your drink.

JENNY: Thank you.

> *(JACK reenters with a platter of fruit and a tray with nuts.)*

THE PROPER TECHNIQUE

JENNY: So tell us about this play you're doing.

JACK: I was just telling Mr. Strauss...

LEO: Leo, please.

JACK: I was just telling Leo that I was thinking of doing The Affairs of Anatol.

JENNY: Ah! Anatol! I played in The Affairs of Anatol, when I was very young. And didn't we do it one summer?

LEO: Very badly.

JENNY: You have a director?

JACK: Not yet.

JENNY: If you're going to do The Affairs Of Anatol, you need someone special. Someone who has heart and someone who knows style. Such a sad, lovely, funny play. *(SHE turns to GEORGE.)* And you'll play Max, of course.

JACK: We haven't thought about casting yet.

JENNY: What an inspired choice!

JACK: You think so?

JENNY: You'll break our hearts. Every woman in the audience. When you start casting I have a couple of young ladies for you to look at. I do some coaching occasionally. There's one young lady who is absolutely amazing. Jack might be interested in sitting in on one of your classes, Leo.

249

THE PROPER TECHNIQUE

LEO: I'm sure that Jack doesn't need my help.

JACK: As a matter of fact I've been thinking about consulting you, though I'm sure you have a tight enough schedule as it is.

JENNY: There's always room for one more.

LEO: Thank you, Mr. Strauss.

JENNY: What did I say? If you can coach that no-talent... I talk too much.

LEO: That's the first accurate statement you've made this evening.

JENNY: My husband is a very modest man. He doesn't realize how important the work he's doing is.

LEO: There are some people who might disagree with you.

JENNY: What was the theatre like before you and our group brought it to life? Declamation. Artificiality.

LEO: *(HE rises and examples the Modigliani.)* I see you're a patron of the arts. Van Gogh is my favorite.

JACK: One of mine as well. I have a magnificent one in my study. Would you care to see it?

LEO: I would love to.

JACK: Follow me.

(THEY go off to the interior.)

250

THE PROPER TECHNIQUE

JENNY: What does it feel like to work for a movie star, when you yourself have talent as well?

GEORGE: Jack's an old friend. We were room mates briefly at Ohio State.

JENNY: Room mates?

GEORGE: Jack was dating his first wife at the time. Eventually they moved in together.

JENNY: I have someone I'd like you to meet. Do you know Rudy Beekman?

GEORGE: Is he an actor?

JENNY: He's a scenic designer. A very talented one.

GEORGE: Oh, yes. I think I've heard of him.

JENNY: He's in town right now, which is unusual, because he's always on the go.

GEORGE: Just a minute. Do you think I'm...homosexual?

JENNY: We don't use that word anymore. The word now is "gay."

GEORGE: Well, if that's what you're thinking. You're quite mistaken, because I don't happen to be...gay.

JENNY: Why are you so touchy? I just thought you might enjoy meeting Rudy.

GEORGE: Why?

THE PROPER TECHNIQUE

JENNY: Because I think that Rudy and you have a great deal in common.

GEORGE: And what might that be?

JENNY: A mental alertness, a wry sort of wit. He's a charming man. If you don't want to meet him, you don't have to.

GEORGE: Let me think about it.

JENNY: Is your boss dating anyone now?

GEORGE: Why? You have someone for him as well?

JENNY: Look, George, I know I'm a busybody. But I mean well. I assure you I do. I like to see people happy. Is that a crime? Do you have any friends here in New York?

GEORGE: Not really, no.

JENNY: I have open house every Friday evening. It sometimes goes on into the wee hours. Come by. You'll meet some people.

GEORGE: Like Rudy Beekman?

JENNY: Rudy shows up sometimes, when he's in town. He travels a lot, to Europe, to London. He has a very interesting life. He designs sets for theatre, for opera.

(The doorbell rings.)

JENNY: Are you expecting someone?

GEORGE: Not that I know of.

THE PROPER TECHNIQUE

JENNY: Then that might be May, my daughter. She said she might drop by if she finished her homework in time. You've met my daughter.

GEORGE: Oh, yes.

(GEORGE opens the door. MAY is discovered.)

MAY: Hello, George. My I come in?

GEORGE: Please do.

MAY: Where is everyone?

JENNY: Everyone is in his study showing your father his Van Gogh. Are you wearing makeup?

MAY: No.

JENNY: Then your cheeks are all flushed.

MAY: Really, Mother.

JENNY: Mother?!

MAY: Jenny.

JENNY: And don't "really" me. *(SHE takes a handkerchief from her bag, moistens it with her tongue, then wipes May's cheek.)* That's rouge.

MAY: Jenny, I'm nineteen years old. Lots of girls my age wear makeup.

THE PROPER TECHNIQUE

JENNY: Lots of girls need makeup. You don't. *(To GEORGE)* Do you think she needs makeup?

MAY: Jenny, please.

JENNY: I'm talking to George here. Do you think my daughter needs makeup? Tell me the truth.

GEORGE: Not really, no.

JENNY: Thank you. From a perfectly objective point of view. You finished your homework?

MAY: Jenny, I'm not in grammar school. And I'm absolutely starved. *(SHE helps herself to the fruit.)*

JENNY: Because you didn't eat dinner.

MAY: I wasn't hungry...then. *(To GEORGE)* May I have a drink?

GEORGE: Would you care for some Moltepuciano?

MAY: You have it?

GEORGE: We made a special point.

JENNY: Oh, you're so sophisticated. Rouge. Moltepuciano.

MAY: When you were nineteen I don't think you were exactly a wallflower.

JENNY: Don't be fresh.

MAY: Do as I say, don't do as I do.

THE PROPER TECHNIQUE

(MAY helps herself to the fruit, while GEORGE pours a glass of wine and places it on the table in front of her.)

MAY: Thank you, George. Do you have any problems with a domineering mother?

JENNY: Wait till you become a mother.

MAY: When and if, I will not be oppressive.

JENNY: *(To GEORGE)* Do you talk to your mother like that?

GEORGE: My mother and I said very little to each other. *(To MAY)* How's the wine?

MAY: *(SHE twirls the glass, smells the bouquet then tastes the wine.)* Not bad.

JENNY: *(Mocking, yet proud)* Oh, she's so continental.

(LEO reenters, followed by JACK.)

LEO: You finished your homework?

MAY: Yes, Daddy, I finished my homework.

(The phone rings. GEORGE answers it.)

GEORGE: Hello? *(HE turns to LEO.)* It's for you, Mr. Strauss.

JENNY: Oh, no!

LEO: *(HE takes the phone.)* Hello? Now calm down, darling. Where are you? How many did you take? Good. Take deep breaths, drink a glass of milk and we'll be right over. *(HE hangs up.)*

JENNY: How many did she take?

LEO: She didn't take any, thank God. I'm sorry, Jack, but we've got to go.

JACK: Yes, of course.

LEO: We'll talk tomorrow. *(To MAY)* You coming with us?

MAY: I just got here.

JACK: We'll put her in a cab.

LEO: I'm sorry to run out on you like this. But that was a student of mine, and she depends on us.

JACK: I hope she's all right.

LEO: It's that system out there on the coast. They don't know how to treat an artist. She's a talented lovely child, and just because she's blonde and sexy they treat her like a piece of meat.

(JENNY kisses GEORGE then JACK.)

JENNY: I told George about my Friday evening open house. Maybe you'll come too.

JACK: Thank you.

JENNY: *(To MAY)* Don't forget. You've got a class tomorrow morning.

THE PROPER TECHNIQUE

MAY: I won't forget.

(GEORGE leads JENNY and LEO off.)

MAY: I wish I had a place of my own. It's awful to be dependent on someone. I resented it, even as a child.

JACK: When did you become an adult?

MAY: Don't you start. How did you and Daddy make out?

JACK: We got along splendidly. As a matter of fact, he's going to work with me. I'm really very excited about it.

MAY: Oh?

JACK: Yes. We're going to work on a scene from The Affairs of Anatol. I'm really very flattered...that he's going to take the time out from, what I'm sure is, a very busy schedule.

MAY: Have you ever studied before?

JACK: Oh, yes. At Ohio State. I took a couple of acting courses. It was laughable though. We just sat around and read a couple of chapters of Stanislavski and that was it. We never took it seriously.

MAY: I see.

JACK: But now, I'm really looking forward to it.

MAY: Are you going to appear in The Affairs of Anatol?

JACK: On Broadway. That's the plan at any rate.

THE PROPER TECHNIQUE

MAY: It's perfect for you.

JACK: You think so?

MAY: Is it all set? I mean, do you have a date and everything?

JACK: It's still in the works. *(After a moment)* You're very lucky, you know.

MAY: In what way?

JACK: To be blessed with a father who's so brilliant.

> *(GEORGE reenters, picks up the empty glasses and goes off.)*

JACK: *(HE sits.)* It's rather frightening, you know. I feel like I'm starting all over again.

MAY: You've been on the stage before.

JACK: As an actor, not as a star. I'm sure the critics will have their little hatchets out for me.

MAY: You do have a lot of fans.

JACK: Fans can be fickle.

MAY: Not all of them.

JACK: You're a strange little creature.

MAY: In what way?

THE PROPER TECHNIQUE

JACK: I don't know. Sometimes I get the impression of a lost little girl.

MAY: And other times?

JACK: A wise old woman.

MAY: Oh.

JACK: That's a compliment.

MAY: Oh.

JACK: You're the kind of daughter I'd like to have had.

MAY: In order to be your daughter, you'd have had to have had me when you were sixteen.

JACK: How do you know how old I am?

MAY: I know lots about you.

JACK: You mean what they print. I'm not really like what you see on the screen.

MAY: Maybe you are, and you don't know it.

JACK: I've always thought that if we ever get to understand our parents, then maybe we'll get to understand ourselves. Do you understand your parents?

MAY: Too well.

JACK: Do you? Really?

THE PROPER TECHNIQUE

MAY: Yes, I think I do.

JACK: Then you must be wise beyond your years. How many beaus to you have?

MAY: I don't have any beaus. I do go out on dates now and then. So far, I haven't found anyone that's really interesting.

JACK: Shallow youth?

MAY: Exactly. Older men are much more interesting.

JACK: By older men you mean...?

MAY: Anyone over thirty.

(GEORGE reenters.)

MAY: If you're cleaning up you can take this as well.

GEORGE: You sure?

MAY: I'm positive.

(GEORGE gathers up the food and goes off.)

MAY: That was thoughtful of you to get the Moltepuciano.

JACK: Nothing's too good for an ardent fan.

MAY: I gather you must like Schnitzler.

JACK: Oh, yes.

THE PROPER TECHNIQUE

MAY: Well, the drama department is doing a Schnitzler play on Friday, and I have an extra ticket. A friend of mine can't make it.

JACK: Not The Affairs Of Anatol?

MAY: No, no. It's La Ronde.

JACK: Why thank you. I would love to see La Ronde.

(GEORGE reenters.)

MAY: I really ought to go. It's a date. Friday night. Can you pick me up at seven?

JACK: Why don't I take you to dinner?

MAY: Would you?

JACK: It would be my pleasure.

MAY: I know of a nice little restaurant near the school.

JACK: I'll pick you up at six. What are you smiling at?

MAY: I can see all my friends when they see me walking in with Jack Gardner.

JACK: We'll put on a show for them.

GEORGE: I'll get a cab. *(HE goes off.)*

MAY: Do you think I ought to try and get a ticket for George as well?

THE PROPER TECHNIQUE

JACK: Let him get his own date.

MAY: But if he's all alone...

JACK: He'll be fine.

MAY: Oh, I forgot. I promised my friend I'd get an autographed picture.

JACK: I didn't bring any with me. I'll send for one.

MAY: Thank you.

(GEORGE reenters.)

GEORGE: Your carriage awaits.

MAY: Thank you. Good night.

JACK: Good night.

(MAY goes off. GEORGE shuts the door.)

GEORGE: You must be out of your mind.

JACK: What?

GEORGE: What?!

JACK: What?

GEORGE: She's just a child.

JACK: Don't be a fool. She's just pleasant company, that's all.

THE PROPER TECHNIQUE

GEORGE: When have I heard that before?

JACK: You're like an old woman.

GEORGE: And you're like a teen-ager.

JACK: Then she and I are perfect for each other.

GEORGE: Suit yourself.

JACK: *(HE pours some wine.)* Would you care for some moltepuciano?

> *(GEORGE doesn't respond. JACK stands at the terrace doors, sipping the wine and looking out over the city.)*

JACK: It is a magical town.

> *(GEORGE sighs and shakes his head as the lights come down.)*

ACT TWO

Scene One

(The following Friday, late afternoon. JACK is discovered seated, in his shirtsleeves, pad and pen in hand. There is a pile of books nearby. GEORGE enters from the outside carrying a handful of books.)

JACK: What have you found?

GEORGE: Two books on the Austro-Hungarian Empire, another biography of Schnitzler, and another translation of The Affairs of Anatol.

JACK: Good god! It's endless.

GEORGE: I don't know why you need all this.

JACK: It's background.

GEORGE: Background for what?

JACK: For Anatol. I told you. Leo wants me to write a biography of Anatol, and how can you write about someone if you don't know his background, how he lived, where he grew up?

GEORGE: How many volumes are you planning on?

JACK: Don't be ridiculous.

GEORGE: I'm not the one that's being ridiculous. You're playing a role. A character that doesn't really exist. How can you write a biography about someone who doesn't exist? Why do you shake your head? All right. I'm superficial, a philistine, an ignoramus. But

THE PROPER TECHNIQUE

I don't see how you can do any acting when your head is full of all that research.

JACK: One step at a time.

GEORGE: Aside from stuffing yourself with all that...research, what exactly have you accomplished? It's been two days now. What have you learned so far?

JACK: *(Reading)* "I was born on the morning of May 15th, 1862."

GEORGE: How do you know that?

JACK: That's when Schnitzler was born. I'm assuming that Anatol is a stand-in for Schnitzler himself.

GEORGE: Why? Why would you assume that Anatol and Schnitzler are one? A character in a play is not necessarily the stand-in for the playwright. Is Othello the stand-in for Shakespeare?

JACK: From what I gather, Anatol is quite similar to Schnitzler. They both had many love affairs.

GEORGE: I see.

JACK: Do you or do you not want to hear what I've got so far?

GEORGE: I'm all ears.

JACK: *(Reading)* "I was born on the morning of May 15th, 1862."

GEORGE: You said that.

THE PROPER TECHNIQUE

JACK: "I was delivered by a midwife." That was the custom in those days. Babies were delivered in the home by a midwife.

GEORGE: Go on.

JACK: That's as far as I've gotten. I'd like to find out the sort of schools young boys attended in those days. I don't know where to look. I assume it was some sort of private school, since Anatol was a wealthy boy.

GEORGE: Lucky Anatol!

JACK: Why are you so cynical?

GEORGE: Why are you so naive? Leo Strauss is a dangerous man. He leaves behind him a string of confused young actors. He takes people apart and neglects to put them together again.

JACK: You think he's taking me apart?

GEORGE: Look. I am not your father. You are an adult, a movie star. You ought to be able to look after yourself; and I say that with some skepticism, since, apparently, you need someone to wipe your ass, and that's one thing I'm not paid to do.

JACK: Tsk, tsk, tsk. Such talk from a well brought up boy from the Midwest.

GEORGE: At least I have the sense I was born with, even though I was delivered in a hospital.

JACK: I am learning things, things I never learned before. It's opened up a whole new world.

THE PROPER TECHNIQUE

GEORGE: It's opened up a hole in your head.

JACK: It gives me more confidence. Don't you understand? Leo Strauss knows that he is doing.

GEORGE: And how long are you going to work on this...epic?

JACK: Until it's finished.

GEORGE: And when might that be?

JACK: When Anatol reaches the age of...I guess around thirty.

GEORGE: Why thirty? Why not forty? Why not seventy?

JACK: Schnitzler died at the age of sixty nine.

GEORGE: And Anatol? That's the character you're writing about. When did Anatol die?

JACK: Don't be ridiculous.

GEORGE: Why am I being ridiculous? If you're so sure you know when he was born, why don't you know when he died?

JACK: Because, as far as I'm concerned, he hasn't died. He's still alive.

GEORGE: Oh, I see. And why do you stop at thirty?

JACK: I think he's about thirty when the play begins.

GEORGE: But you're not really sure.

THE PROPER TECHNIQUE

JACK: All right, George. Scoff if you like. But when I get up on that stage and give an absolutely brilliant performance...

GEORGE: I pray to God.

JACK: You know what your problem is?

GEORGE: No, but I know you're going to tell me.

JACK: You have no...sense of dedication.

GEORGE: Thank God. I thought you were going to tell me I'm a ham.

JACK: I wouldn't do that. And do you know why?

GEORGE: Why?

JACK: Because I happen to be considerate and supportive...a word, apparently, you are unacquainted with. I mean, the critics are out there with their knives. I need all the help, all the support I can get.

(*The doorbell rings.*)

JACK: That must be Leo.

GEORGE: You're working here?

JACK: Jenny has her Friday get-to-gethers, and she takes over the whole house, including his studio.

(*The doorbell rings again.*)

JACK: Are you going to open the door, or shall I?

THE PROPER TECHNIQUE

GEORGE: Anatol, please, you're not old enough to get out of the cradle.

(GEORGE opens the door and admits LEO.)

LEO: Good afternoon.

GEORGE: Good afternoon.

LEO: Jenny's expecting you, you know.

GEORGE: Yes, I know.

LEO: You're not going to disappoint her?

GEORGE: How many people attend these soirees of hers?

LEO: It's a mob scene. I always try to find an excuse to escape. In your case, however, it would give you an opportunity to meet people since, I gather you don't have many friends in town.

GEORGE: Do you know who she's expecting?

LEO: One never knows who's going to turn up. Sometimes it's a foreign dignitary, a writer, a director and actors by the dozen.

GEORGE: Rudy Beekman?

LEO: You know Rudy?

GEORGE: Jenny wanted me to meet him.

LEO: I see. Yes, I think you two should hit it off.

269

THE PROPER TECHNIQUE

GEORGE: Why do you say that?

LEO: Rudy's very quick, very bright...and very talented. I think you'd like Rudy. *(HE turns to JACK.)* So, how's it coming?

JACK: Very slowly. There's so much material.

LEO: Well, we can put that aside for now.

JACK: I've barely started...

LEO: You can finish it at your leisure.

JACK: George?

GEORGE: Yes? What is it?

JACK: Are you staying or are you going?

GEORGE: I'm sorry. I didn't mean to hold up progress. I'll see you in the morning. *(HE goes off.)*

LEO: So, let's get started.

JACK: I'm not used to delving into a character like this. My mind works rather quickly and I usually go by my instinct. As a matter of fact, I've often found analysis rather stultifying.

LEO: Who have you studied with?

JACK: No one, to speak of. Our instructor at Ohio State, was not very forthcoming. We did scenes and he critiqued them, and that was it.

THE PROPER TECHNIQUE

LEO: They had a drama department?

JACK: If you can call it that. I was sorry, afterward, that I didn't go to Yale or Harvard. I've looked over the scene you suggested. Would you like to start with that?

LEO: We'll get to that eventually. I'd like to start with some exercises first.

JACK: Okay. I must warn you. I'm not very good at this sort of thing.

LEO: Have you tried it?

JACK: Well, we did get to do some improvisations.

LEO: That's quite all right. You're all tensed up. Why don't we take it one step at a time. Actually, I'll be encapsulating work that I usually spread out over a matter of weeks, sometimes months.

JACK: Do you think that's wise?

LEO: In your case, with your background, I think it's permissible.

JACK: There is no deadline, you know. What I mean to say is, I'm not going to face that mob out there, that may want my head, until I'm absolutely ready.

LEO: I can see you're very tense. I want you to relax.

JACK: How do I do that?

> (*LEO takes a chair and places it in the middle of the room.*)

THE PROPER TECHNIQUE

LEO: Sit down. Let your arms hang loose. I can see the tension here, right here. (*HE touches Jack's forehead just above the nose.*) You don't mind if I touch you?

JACK: No, no, no. That's quite all right.

LEO: And here at the side of your nose. Relax. Make your mind a blank. I can see the tension here, in the back of the neck. (*HE places his hands there and massages JACK.*) You're tied up in knots. Relax. Your mind is an open book. The body is an instrument, waiting to be played. Open. Receptive.

JACK: I really am tensed up.

LEO: Sometimes making noises helps one to relax.

JACK: What kind of noises?

LEO: Any kind of noises. Just let it out.

> (*JACK starts to howl and grunt and make all sorts of noises.*)

LEO: Fine. That's fine.

JACK: (*JACK heaves a sigh.*) That felt good.

LEO: Good.

JACK: Where do we go from here?

LEO: Let's do an exercise in sense memory. The ability to focus is very important. I would like you to get up, walk over to that table, pick up a book, walk back to the chair, sit down, and leaf through the pages of the book and then set it down.

JACK: Should I look for something specific?

LEO: You might do that.

JACK: I'll look up Schnitzler, education. How's that?

LEO: Fine.

JACK: Or do you think that's too specific?

LEO: I'll leave that up to you.

JACK: Shall I start now?

LEO: Whenever you're ready.

> *(JACK rises, picks up the book, returns to the chair and leafs through the book and sets it down.)*

JACK: I looked up education, but I didn't find anything.

LEO: That's quite all right. Now, I want you to return the book, go back to your seat, and I want you to repeat the same action from memory without using the book.

JACK: You want me to pantomime?

LEO: *(Nods)* I want you to focus on remembering what you did. I want you to duplicate that action from memory.

JACK: Right. *(JACK sighs, hangs his arms loosely and rolls his head around to relax, then mimes the action.)* It was a little different I think. Shall I try it again?

LEO: No, no, no. What do you think you learned from that exercise?

JACK: What was I supposed to learn?

LEO: Your mind, your body was fully intent on that one action. You were focused. You were relaxed and you were focused.

JACK: Then that was good, wasn't it?

LEO: *(HE nods patiently.)* Now, let's try an improvisation. Anatol gets up in the morning. It's the morning of his wedding. He goes through his regular morning ritual, shaving, etcetera, and then getting dressed. All the while he's thinking. He loves the girl he's going to marry, but then he remembers the girl he just broke off with. He loved her, too. Should he have broken off with her? Is this wedding a mistake he'll regret for the rest of his life?

JACK: And what does he decide?

LEO: I'll leave that up to you. Take your time. And when you start I want you to be specific. I want you to concentrate. I want you to focus on what you are doing.

JACK: And I'm dealing with this problem, this mental problem. Or is it an emotional problem?

LEO: What do you think?

JACK: I think it's both.

THE PROPER TECHNIQUE

LEO: A very interesting deduction. The mind governs the emotion.

JACK: So actually there are three things going on at the same time. I mean the mental and emotional turmoil, that's two things and then there's the ablutions. *(HE looks perplexed.)*

LEO: Yes? What is it?

JACK: Well, there are a number of questions to be answered. For one thing... Do you think Anatol has a mustache or a goatee? Or both? What was the style in those days?

LEO: For the sake of the exercise, let's assume he has neither.

JACK: That'll make it easier.

LEO: Is there anything else?

JACK: Well, I assume Anatol shaved with a straight razor, and he had a basin into which he poured the water...

LEO: Anything else?

JACK: He probably used a shaving soap and a brush which I'm unfamiliar with.

LEO: All right. Let's change the situation. You, Jack Gardner, are in that same ticklish situation. You're getting married, but you're still in love with the girl you broke off with.

JACK: That sure hits home.

LEO: Good, good.

THE PROPER TECHNIQUE

JACK: That's rather a sore point at the moment. Can we go somewhere else? May I ask where all this is leading? What's the purpose of all these exercises?

LEO: I'm glad you asked. It's the easiest thing in the world to follow one's instincts and give a brilliant performance on opening night. But what about the day after, and the day after that? How can we duplicate what was so brilliant the day before?

JACK: Would we want to...duplicate it? What I mean to say...

LEO: Maybe duplicate is not the right word. We want to keep our performance fresh, day after day, week after week....hopefully.

JACK: Yes, hopefully. Oh, I agree with you there. It wasn't easy keeping it fresh.

LEO: You've had that problem before?

JACK: Oh, yes. I toured for eight months in Darkness At Noon. I learned more about acting in those eight months.

LEO: Good, good. Then you know how valuable it is to keep things fresh.

JACK: Oh, indeed I do.

LEO: Then I think it's time to move on. I think it's time now to get to the heart of the program.

JACK: And what might that be?

LEO: Affective memory. I want you to go back into the past. I want you to remember a personal moment in your life, an emotional moment, a painful moment, one that made a deep impression. Take your time. There's no rush.

JACK: *(After a few moments)* Well...

LEO: No, no, no. I don't want you to tell me what it was. I just want you to recreate that moment. Take your time. Start whenever you're ready.

JACK: It doesn't matter what kind of a moment it was?

LEO: As long as it was personal and painful.

JACK: Okay.

LEO: Take your time.

> *(JACK sits thoughtfully, then places the chair some feet back and sits down. HE becomes grief-stricken. After a moment he rises slowly, walks forward and looks down. HE is shaken and walks back to his seat. After a while he rises, walks around the room, then stands with his back to Leo, looking up at something a few yards away. Suddenly HE crumbles and breaks down sobbing.)*

LEO: That was fine.

> *(JACK continues to sob. HE sobs uncontrollably. After a long while he gains control. LEO hands him his handkerchief.)*

JACK: Thank you. I'm sorry.

LEO: No, no, no. That was fine. May I ask what occurred?

THE PROPER TECHNIQUE

JACK: I had a younger sister. She died rather suddenly. At the funeral home I sat in the back, but then, after a while, I gathered up my courage and I walked up to the casket, and I looked down at her lying there pale and lifeless, and I almost passed out. And then, later, when we proceeded to the cemetery, and she was lowered into the grave, I stood quite a few yards away. I couldn't bear to be too close. And then suddenly I started to sob, and I just couldn't stop. An aunt of mine put her arm around my shoulder, but I just kept on sobbing.

LEO: I'm sure that will be a very useful moment to call up.

JACK: I don't think I could ever go there again, not while I'm on stage at any rate.

LEO: Well, of course, you won't live the moment again, but you'll remember the pain.

JACK: It would tear me apart. I really don't think that's a good idea.

(The phone rings.)

LEO: You relax. I'll take it. *(HE picks up the phone.)* Hello? Yes, dear. When did that happen? Now, listen, Honey... Hold on for one minute. *(HE turns to Jack.)* Do you mind if I take this in your study? It's very important.

JACK: No. No, of course. Go right ahead.

(LEO sets down the phone and goes off to the interior. JACK rises, goes to the bar and shakily pours himself a drink. HE then goes to the phone, puts it to his ear then gently hangs up. HE sits nursing his drink. The doorbell

rings. HE sets down the glass and opens the door. MAY is discovered.)

MAY: I hope I'm not interrupting.

JACK: No, no, no. Come on in.

MAY: You look awful. What's happened?

JACK: Don't ask.

MAY: Is it serious?

JACK: It was once. It still is, I guess. Wow!

MAY: Is Daddy still here?

JACK: He's in the study, on the phone with Marilyn.

MAY: Have you been working with him?

JACK: In spades.

MAY: You've been working on affective memory.

JACK: How do you know?

MAY: I don't know why you wanted to work with him in the first place.

JACK: I'm a coward, I guess. I'm just terrified about facing a Broadway audience.

THE PROPER TECHNIQUE

MAY: That's why I gave it up. Daddy thought I was hopeless anyway. Why do you want to come back to Broadway?

JACK: I was most alive when I was on the stage. Oh, I enjoy acting in the movies. It's very gratifying, but I miss that contact with an audience, the immediate response. I watch one of my movies in the theatre and I hear the audience laughing, but they're not laughing at me. They're laughing at that guy up there on the screen.

MAY: It's natural to be nervous. Helen Hayes throws up on opening night. Laurence Olivier, for years, suffered with stage fright.

JACK: Did he really?

MAY: And that's Laurence Olivier.

JACK: That is sort of reassuring, isn't it? I'm afraid I'm a great disappointment to your father. I don't think I did well on those exercises he gave me.

MAY: I wouldn't worry about it.

JACK: He may not want to continue to work with me.

MAY: Daddy isn't for everyone, you know.

JACK: I'm sure he doesn't need the money, but I am prepared to pay him well.

MAY: I'm sure it's not a matter of money. Have you finished for the day?

THE PROPER TECHNIQUE

JACK: I'm not quite sure.

MAY: It is almost five, and I was in the area and I thought it was pointless for me to go back home. I thought we might go directly to the restaurant from here. Besides, if you did pick me up at home you'd run into Jenny's open house, and I don't think you'd want to do that. I knew you were working with Daddy, and I thought I could always wait in the lobby.

JACK: There's no need for you to do that. Can I offer you some wine?

MAY: That might be nice. Thank you.

JACK: *(HE pours some wine.)* That's a very pretty dress.

MAY: Thank you.

JACK: Have you done something to your hair?

MAY: Why do you ask?

JACK: I don't know. You look different somehow.

MAY: Do I?

(HE hands her the wine.)

MAY: Thank you. Aren't you going to join me.

JACK: I'd better wait and see if we're going to continue. How was your day?

THE PROPER TECHNIQUE

MAY: It was okay.

(*LEO reenters.*)

LEO: What are you doing here?

JACK: She's come to pick me up. After we're through that is.

LEO: Oh?

JACK: We're going to see La Ronde. It's being done by the Drama Department.

LEO: I see.

JACK: Shall we continue?

LEO: What's that? No, no, no. I think we've done enough for today.

JACK: Can I offer you a drink? It's Scotch on the rocks. Only I don't have any ice at the moment.

LEO: That's quite all right. I'll take it straight.

JACK: One Scotch coming up. (*HE pours a drink.*) I'm afraid I didn't do very well.

(*There is an obvious silence on the part of LEO. JACK hands him the drink.*)

LEO: Thank you.

THE PROPER TECHNIQUE

JACK: Would you mind entertaining each other while I change? May and I are going to dinner before the theatre.

LEO: I see.

JACK: Excuse me. *(HE goes off.)*

LEO: What is this?

MAY: What?

LEO: What?! This man is twice your age.

MAY: Not quite.

LEO: What do you mean not quite?

MAY: He's one year shy.

LEO: Don't be clever with me.

MAY: I'm not being clever. I'm just stating a fact.

LEO: I don't want you dating him.

MAY: Why?

LEO: For one thing, he's too old.

MAY: As a matter of fact, in many ways I think he's much younger than I am.

LEO: You heard what I said.

THE PROPER TECHNIQUE

MAY: What have you got against him?

LEO: He's a phony, a Hollywood phony.

MAY: Now you know that isn't true. He's charming and amiable...

LEO: From your point of view, perhaps.

MAY: And from your point of view?

LEO: He's a vicious, nasty man, and he has contempt for everything that I stand for.

MAY: Daddy, what are you talking about? Didn't he ask to study with you?

LEO: Only to make fun of me. I was doing my best to help him, and he was laughing at me. I could tell. He was laughing at me all the time.

MAY: I don't think so, Daddy.

LEO: You don't think so. You know so much. In your nineteen years you've acquired the wisdom of a Minerva.

MAY: Living with you and Jenny has taught me a lot.

LEO: What is that supposed to mean? Is that one of your sarcastic observations?

MAY: Why are you so sensitive?

LEO: The question is, Why are you so insensitive? I don't know

284

where you came from. Not from me certainly, and not from your mother. You have no respect for our feelings or for our work.

MAY: That isn't true.

LEO: I don't want you seeing him anymore. Did you hear what I said? He was sitting there laughing at me.

MAY: I think you're mistaken, Daddy. He has great respect for you.

LEO: Is that what he told you?

MAY: Yes.

LEO: And you believe him?

MAY: Why should he lie about a thing like that?

LEO: I'll tell you why. Because he wants to get into your pants, that's why. He's a lecher. A cradle robber. He's been married twice, you know.

MAY: Two demerits.

LEO: We've been too easy with you. That's the trouble. And the fault is mine. I'll admit it. I have a lot on my mind, and your mother is too...indulgent. You are still a virgin, aren't you?

MAY: Unfortunately. All my friends have had, at least, one affair.

LEO: I'm not saying that you have to go through life a spinster, but when you do make love, it should be with the right man. I'm sure your mother told you that. Does she know you're going out with him?

(MAY nods.)

LEO: And she approves?

(MAY nods.)

LEO: Are you telling me the truth?

MAY: You're going to ask her anyway.

LEO: Your mother and I are going to have a long, long talk.

MAY: Oh God, no!

(JACK reenters wearing a tie and a jacket.)

JACK: Well, I'm all set. We're going to dinner, Leo, and then the theatre. The Drama Department at the University is doing La Ronde.

LEO: Are they really?

JACK: I don't suppose you'd care to join us.

(MAY tries to signal JACK in the negative.)

LEO: As a matter of fact, that's a great idea. Friday night in our house is chaotic.

MAY: We're going to the Bistro for dinner, you know. You hate the food there.

THE PROPER TECHNIQUE

LEO: I'm sure I can find something on the menu.

MAY: And I'm sure the show's sold out. They always do sell out.

LEO: I'm sure they can find a seat for me. And I would love to hear about our friend here's experience in Lotus Land. I'll go round up a cab. *(HE goes off.)*

MAY: Why did you invite him?

JACK: I thought it was the thing to do. And besides, if we're going to work together, I think we ought to get to know each other better.

MAY: Jack...

JACK: What?

MAY: You are not going to be working together.

JACK: Oh?

MAY: Daddy thinks you've been making fun of him.

JACK: Why in the world would he think that?

MAY: Daddy's really very insecure.

JACK: Is he really?

MAY: Once you get to know him. His method has come under attack, you know.

THE PROPER TECHNIQUE

JACK: I'll try to remember that. I certainly wouldn't want to alienate him. If I say the wrong thing, please, please stop me.

MAY: I'm afraid it may be too late.

(The door is opened by LEO.)

LEO: The cab is here. Come along, come along.

(LEO comes into the room and ushers MAY and JACK out the door as the lights come down.)

Scene Two

(The following Monday, late morning. The room is empty. The phone rings for quite some time. GEORGE enters from the interior and picks up the phone.)

GEORGE: Hello? Oh, hi, Rudy. I just got up, and I was just about to call you. It was a wonderful day. All right, A magnificent day. This evening? No. What would you like to do? Are you a good cook? Really? You have all sorts of talents. No, I have no plans for the summer. No, I've never been to Fire Island. Well, I don't know. No, I'd love to. I really would. Let me talk to Jack. I'd have to give him some sort of notice. No, no, no. we're just friends. Today's paper? What about it? I never read the gossip columns. What does Liz Smith have to say? Oh, dear. He must be out of his mind. Read it to me again. Don't get me wrong. I think she's very sweet, but she's half his age...in years, at any rate. It's amazing. For a man his age, and his experience, he's really very naive, and very vulnerable. All right, all right. I'll see you at six.

(GEORGE hangs up and sits lost in thought. JACK enters from the outside, accompanied by MAY. HE carries two overnight bags.)

JACK: Good morning!

GEORGE: Well, you seem bright and chipper.

JACK: Why shouldn't I be? The sun is shining, and all's right with the world.

MAY: Good morning, George.

GEORGE: Good morning.

MAY: *(In a bass voice, imitating him.)* Good morning.

289

THE PROPER TECHNIQUE

GEORGE: Obviously the week-end agreed with the two of you.

JACK: It was a glorious week-end. We went swimming, we went sailing. We dined and we danced. We danced and we dined. Didn't we, Miss Strauss?

MAY: We most certainly did.

JACK: And I'm here to announce that the Hamptons is a glorious place to spend the week-end.

GEORGE: I didn't know you were spending the week-end together.

JACK: You don't approve.

GEORGE: I'm not the girl's father and, incidentally, it might interest you to know that the two of you have made the gossip columns.

JACK: Oh, dear.

MAY: Which column is that?

GEORGE: Liz Smith.

MAY: What did she write?

GEORGE: "What daughter of a famous acting guru has been seen with what movie idol twice her age?"

JACK: Ah, well.

GEORGE: "Is romance in the air?" I assume your parents are aware of all this.

THE PROPER TECHNIQUE

JACK: Well, Jenny did send us off with her blessing, didn't she?

GEORGE: And your father? Did he send you off with his blessing? You're not twenty one, you know. *(HE starts off, then stops.)* Oh, and, incidentally.....

JACK: Yes?

GEORGE: What's that?

JACK: You were about to say something.

GEORGE: Yes, well, I'd better get started on the mail. *(HE goes off.)*

JACK: Something's come over George.

MAY: Oh?

JACK: I don't know what happened at that open house of your mother's on Friday, but Saturday morning George Butterworth was a completely different person.

MAY: In what way?

JACK: He seemed happy.

MAY: Is that so unusual?

JACK: George can be sarcastic. He can be witty, he can be nasty, but I have never seen him happy.

MAY: When I got home Friday night, the open house was still in full swing, and George was sitting with Rudy Beekman, chattering away, and he certainly seemed happy to me.

JACK: That's interesting. I wonder if George has finally...

MAY: What?

JACK: Never mind. I made up my mind, years ago, that I would never pry into George's personal life. Since then we've gotten along splendidly. Of course, that hasn't prevented him from sticking his nose into my affairs. Come to think of it, I don't think George has had a personal life...up until now I suspect. *(HE takes her hand.)* You tired?

MAY: No. I'm wide awake.

(THEY sit, snuggle and kiss.)

JACK: So, what shall I do?

MAY: About what?

JACK: About the play. I really am torn. I don't want to make a fool of myself, and I've really been looking forward to getting back on the stage. The trouble is I'm not just another actor now, I'm a movie star and, of course, that may sell some tickets, but then I've got all this weight to carry, a responsibility I'm not quite ready to take on.

MAY: Well, if you're really that insecure, I would wait.

JACK: And then what?

THE PROPER TECHNIQUE

MAY: I'd find some out-of-the-way theatre and try the play out there.

JACK: Now why didn't I think of that?

MAY: I mean, if you were a boxer, even if you had won a number of fights, you would still go into training, wouldn't you?

JACK: Where did you learn all this?

MAY: I didn't learn anything. It's just a matter of common sense.

JACK: Common sense is rarely common. As a matter of fact, a few years ago this little theatre out in San Bernardino invited me to do a play there. I'm sure they'd be happy to have me.

MAY: Are they still functioning?

JACK: Not only functioning, they seem to be thriving. As a matter of fact, there are several theatres out on the coast, little theatres that have done some rather interesting work. How did I ever manage without you? You hungry, because I'm absolutely starved. I did have a menu somewhere. Ah, here it is. (*HE hands her the menu.*)

MAY: I'm really not very hungry.

JACK: Well, it is lunch time, and we didn't have much of a breakfast.

MAY: I'll have a tuna fish sandwich and a lobster bisque. Just a cup.

JACK: Sounds good to me. (*HE picks up the phone and dials.*) Ah,

293

THE PROPER TECHNIQUE

Henry. It's Jack Gardner. Can you send up two tuna fish sandwiches and two cups of lobster bisque. That's quite all right. *(HE hangs up.)* If we do decide to go to the coast, what about school?

MAY: What?

JACK: I said...

MAY: Yes, yes, I heard you.

JACK: You seem preoccupied.

MAY: Well, the fact of the matter is, school is the least of my worries.

JACK: Oh?

MAY: It's Daddy, Jack. He hates you.

JACK: He hates me? Friday night at dinner, and when we were at the theatre he was absolutely charming. Why in the world would your father hate me?

MAY: I told you, Jack. He thinks you've been making fun of him...when he was working with you on those exercises.

JACK: Well, that's ridiculous. I did everything he told me to do. I did have a question or two because I wanted to make sure I did everything right, but I certainly wasn't trying to make fun of him. Well, I'm sorry if he misunderstood. Is he home right now, do you think?

MAY: He does have a class this afternoon, I know.

THE PROPER TECHNIQUE

(JACK goes to the phone, consults a note pad, picks up the phone and dials.)

MAY: And he never answers the phone.

(The door is thrown up and LEO enters. JACK hangs up.)

LEO: So...there you are! Has he touched you?

MAY: Daddy...

JACK: Leo...

LEO: And you, you son of a bitch, I'll kill you.

JACK: You're not gonna kill me, Leo, unless... You're not concealing a gun, are you?

LEO: *(To MAY)* I'll deal with you later. Which bag is yours?

JACK: Leo, will you please calm down?

LEO: She's coming home with me, and if you ever come around our house again I'll call the cops. *(HE grabs a bag.)*

JACK: That's my bag.

(LEO drops the bag and picks up the other one.)

MAY: Daddy, you're being ridiculous.

LEO: Sneaking off like that, without even a word. Liebchen, how could you do this to me?

THE PROPER TECHNIQUE

MAY: I didn't sneak off. I spoke to Jenny about it, and she gave us her blessing.

LEO: Who is the head of our household, me or your mother?

MAY: That's a matter of opinion.

LEO: You got a fresh tongue, kid. You know that?

MAY: Daddy, Jack and I are in love.

LEO: Love?! What do you know about love? You can't even wipe your nose.

JACK: Leo, we spent a perfectly harmless week-end together, in separate rooms.

LEO: Did you really? Well, now, that's very interesting and, come to think of it, that makes a lot of sense.

JACK: What do you mean?

LEO: You know what I mean, Mister Pantywaist. *(HE turns to MAY.)* Your friend here is a pervert.

JACK: What are you talking about?

LEO: You know what I'm talking about. You and that...so-called secretary of yours.

JACK: What? You think I'm gay?

LEO: I wasn't born yesterday, mister.

THE PROPER TECHNIQUE

JACK: I hate to disillusion you, Leo.

LEO: The next thing you're going to tell me that George isn't gay.

JACK: Think about it, Leo. If I were gay, why would I come on to your daughter?

LEO: All right, so you swing both ways? Is that the kind of man you want, my child?

JACK: Actually, Leo, I'm glad you brought that up.

LEO: What?

JACK: I didn't want to offend you, but I have been concerned about this little problem you seem to be having.

LEO: Problem? What are you talking about?

JACK: "You don't mind if I touch you, do you?'

LEO: What?

JACK: During those so-called exercises of yours, isn't that what you said, as you placed your hands gently on my face, and then moved on to the back of my neck.

LEO: What? Are you crazy?

JACK: Maybe you're not aware of it, Leo. Maybe it's something you've been fighting all your life. That's not uncommon now, is it?

LEO: You think you're so clever.

THE PROPER TECHNIQUE

(JENNY enters through the open doorway slamming the door closed behind her.)

LEO: Aha, the traitor! The traitor who sold her daughter for a pound of flesh.

JENNY: He thinks he's back on the stage. For one thing, my dear, you never played Shylock. In addition to that, you were a lousy actor to begin with.

LEO: I was a lousy actor? Ha!

JENNY: At least I happened to have had a career, before I married you, that is.

LEO: A career? You sang in that little revue of yours, and very badly I might add. And you danced a little. I won't even comment on that.

JENNY: And what did you do? Walk-ons, forgettable parts in forgettable plays?

LEO: What I did is not important. And what you did is of even less importance. What's important is the fate of our daughter.
(HE approaches MAY tearfully and takes her head in his hands.)
Darling, baby, I had such hopes for you, such hopes.

MAY: Oh, Daddy, I am not an actress. I never was and I never will be.

JENNY: Oh, for God's sake, Leo, stop already.

LEO: You, you traitor! You I lost faith in a long time ago.

THE PROPER TECHNIQUE

JENNY: Me? You talk to me about losing faith? You adulterer!

LEO: Me you're calling an adulterer?

JENNY: Once! Just once.

LEO: Aha!

JENNY: And I had a miserable time. And would you like me to go down the list?

LEO: There is no list. And I don't think we have to go through all of this in front of the child.

JENNY: What child? If you're referring to my daughter, she happens to have more sense than the both of us put together.

LEO: All right. Let's stop this foolishness. Come. Let's go home. We'll talk about this at dinner, when we can sit down and talk calmly.

JACK: Leo, May and I are going to be married, if your daughter will have me, that is.

MAY: And she will.

JACK: And we would like your consent.

LEO: Married? She's still a baby. Where do you think this is, Russia?

(The door bell rings.)

THE PROPER TECHNIQUE

JACK: That must be our lunch. Is anyone hungry? I can order you something? Leo? Jenny? The food here's quite good.

(JACK opens the door, takes the tray, mutters "Thanks" then closes the door and places the tray on a table.)

MAY: Mmmm, that looks good.. *(SHE sits down.)* We had a wonderful week-end. *(SHE starts on the soup.)*

LEO: I don't want to hear about it.

JACK: For your information, we did not make love. *(HE sits down next to MAY.)*

LEO: So you said.

JACK: I guess I'm old fashioned, Leo. I'd like to wait until we're married. *(HE starts on his soup.)*

(LEO looks at JENNY.)

JENNY: You heard what he said.

LEO: All right. I was mistaken.

JACK: Your apology is accepted. This soup's very good. Would you like me to order some for you?

LEO: Let's sit down and talk this over like sensible people.

JENNY: Leo, give it up.

LEO: All right, all right. Of course, you'll wait until after the opening.

THE PROPER TECHNIQUE

JACK: As a matter if fact, there's been a change of plans. I've decided to postpone my Broadway debut.

LEO: A very wise move. We've got a lot of work to do. I know you have a low opinion of me.

JACK: That's not true, Leo. I have the greatest respect for you.

JENNY: Leo, no one's questioning your work

LEO: My work is controversial. I know that. But you talk to some of the biggest stars in Hollywood. You talk to all those people who have studied with me, all those people who are thankful for what I've done for them.

JENNY: All right, already. You're a genius.

JACK: The fact of the matter is, I've come to the conclusion that I've got to find my own way. Actually I did quite well the last time I appeared on the stage. I'm sure it will all come back to me. May suggested I find an out-of-the-way theatre and start out there. And then, when and if I'm ready, I'll come back and make my Broadway debut.

LEO: A very wise decision.

JACK: I'm glad you think so, Leo. There's this little theatre out on the coast.

LEO: The coast? *(To MAY)* You're going to the coast?

MAY: I guess so.

LEO: *(To JENNY)* They're going to the coast?

THE PROPER TECHNIQUE

JENNY: You'll have the wedding here, of course.

JACK: And as soon as possible.

LEO: What about school?

MAY: The term's over in two weeks.

LEO: You're not going back? You're finished studying? You know everything already?

MAY: If I want to continue to study, there are lots of universities out there, Daddy.

LEO: She's going to the coast?

JENNY: Yes, she's going to the coast. They have planes now, Leo. They fly back and forth, every day now.

(GEORGE enters.)

GEORGE: I thought I heard voices.

JENNY: George, my dear, what's this I hear?

GEORGE: What?

JENNY: You and Rudy. I talked to Rudy this morning.

GEORGE: Yes...well, it's true. Rudy and I...have...hit it off.

JENNY: And you have me to thank.

THE PROPER TECHNIQUE

GEORGE: Yes, I do. Thank you, Jenny. And now that you've brought it up, I...ah... I do have an announcement to make.

LEO: An announcement? What sort of announcement?

GEORGE: Actually it was Rudy's idea. As a matter of fact, he insisted.

LEO: So let's hear the announcement.

GEORGE: This may come as quite a schock.

LEO: All right, already.

GEORGE: As a matter of fact, in a manner of speaking...

LEO: So let's hear it already.

GEORGE: Well, the fact of the matter is...I am...gay.

LEO: That's the announcement? My daughter's getting married. Now that's an announcement.

GEORGE: I'm very happy for you, Jack. *(HE hesitates, then embraces him.)*

JACK: Thank you.

GEORGE: Congratulations. *(HE kisses MAY.)*

MAY: Thank you, George.

JACK: I think this calls for a toast. Jenny, what can I get you?

THE PROPER TECHNIQUE

JENNY: It's kind of early in the day.

JACK: It's never too early to celebrate a happy ending. *(HE pours the drinks.)* A Grand Marnier for Jenny. Leo, Scotch. For the blushing bride.

MAY & JACK: Moltepuciano

JACK: And George?

GEORGE: The wine of choice, of course.

JACK: And, the same for yours truly.

GEORGE: To the happy couple.

JENNY: Couples.

JACK: Moltepuciano!

EVERYONE: *(Standing and raising their glasses)* Moltepuciano!

> *(A lively Italian love song is heard and, as the lights come down, THEY drink.)*

POLITICS AS USUAL
A Play In One Act

CAST OF CHARACTERS
Helen Abrams Whitlock
Andrew Whitlock
Neil Grady

SCENE
A spacious apartment on Central Park West in New
York City

(Late afternoon. The living room of a spacious apartment on Central Park West in New York City. HELEN WHITLOCK, a striking looking woman in her late thirties, enters from the foyer. SHE wears a very stylish suit and is carrying a suitcase. SHE looks about.)

HELEN: Andy? *(SHE sets down the suitcase and goes to the doorway leading to the interior.)* Andy? *(SHE shrugs, sighs and starts to pour some Scotch, then stops.)* No, no! *(SHE pours herself a soft drink, sits with a sigh and sips her soda. After a moment, SHE sets down the glass, goes to the phone and dials.)* Jeb, it's me. Yes, I'm back. Is Andy there? Oh? Have you any idea where he is? The Senate's not in session, is it? I didn't think so. Is everything all right? Oh, well, I'm sure he'll show up eventually. Thank you, dear.

(As HELEN hangs up, ANDY WHITLOCK, wearing a shirt, trousers and slippers, enters from the interior. He is a dapper man in his late thirties.)

ANDY: You're back!

HELEN: Where were you?

ANDY: In the shower. Ohhhhhhh.

HELEN: Yes. I step off the plane...and where is my beau? Where is my beautiful bouquet of red roses?

ANDY: I lost track of the time.

HELEN: Are you all right?

ANDY: *(HE rushes to her and smothers her with kisses.)* I missed you so. Did you miss me?

HELEN: When I had the time. No hubby, no flowers.

ANDY: Am I forgiven?

HELEN: I'll take it under consideration.

ANDY: I've driven you to drink.

HELEN: You flatter yourself. That's ginger ale.

ANDY: You look fabulous.

HELEN: "You lost track of the time."

ANDY: Mea culpa. No, I mean it. You look extra special. You glow.

HELEN: Oh, really!

ANDY: How was the trip?

HELEN: Exhausting.

ANDY: Tell me. Tell me everything. Did you accomplish anything?

HELEN: It's hard to say. You go, expecting to change the world, and then you're confronted with attitudes, attitudes formed by centuries of conflict. And, as a Jew, I hate to admit it, but some of the Israelis, the religious fanatics, they're just as bad, or even worse than the Arabs.

ANDY: And Howard?

HELEN: I've worked for Howard...how long has it been now? Good Lord, it's been thirteen years, and my respect for him continues to grow. He's a warrior, and he was charm personified.

ANDY: I'm jealous.

HELEN: On the other hand...

ANDY: What?

HELEN: He's not nearly as sexy as you are.

ANDY: How do you know?

HELEN: He's a happily married man, and so am I...a married woman, who's no longer irresistible. And a woman, I'll have you know, with some very exciting news.

ANDY: You got a raise.

HELEN: Perish the thought.

ANDY: You've been promoted.

(SHE shakes her head.)

ANDY: Is it a secret?

HELEN: Not for very long.

ANDY: What?

HELEN: You're going to be a father.

ANDY: Who's the mother?

HELEN: *(SHE hits him.)* Aren't you excited?

ANDY: Yes, of course, I am. *(HE kisses her.)* You're going to make a lovely mother.

HELEN: We were looking forward to it, weren't we?.

ANDY: Yes, of course, we were. I'm excited, I really am. So that's why there's no martini.

(SHE eyes him suspiciously.)

ANDY: What? What is it?

HELEN: Andy?!.

ANDY: I'm excited. I really am.

HELEN: Andy! There is something wrong. What is it?

ANDY: You're gonna hate me. You know I love you. I love you so much...

HELEN: Cut the bullshit!

POLITICS AS USUAL

(HE pretends to be shocked.)

HELEN: Now tell me. What is it?

ANDY: I love you so much...

HELEN: So you've said.

ANDY: That when you're not here...

HELEN: When I'm not here...

ANDY: I miss you terribly.

HELEN: Is that all?

ANDY: The fact of the matter is, you know that I'm a twitter freak.

HELEN: Go on!

ANDY: You know that I used to get on the internet...and...

HELEN: I'm listening.

ANDY: When you're not here...when I'm here, all alone...I get so...needy.

HELEN: You mean horny.

ANDY: Yes, horny.

HELEN: And?

POLITICS AS USUAL

ANDY: Yes, well...you see...

HELEN: I'm listening.

ANDY: It's just that... these pictures that I sent...

HELEN: Pictures? What sort of Pictures?

ANDY: Pictures of myself...in a state of...in a state of excitement.

HELEN: You mean...with an erection?

ANDY: Well, yes.

HELEN: I see. And you sent these pictures of yourself to some women...with an erection...over the internet? Is that it? Go on.

ANDY: Well, apparently someone's been hacking into my Email, and this morning, they're all over the place. I mean the pictures...

HELEN: Of yourself with an erection.

ANDY: And some of the messages.

HELEN: What sort of messages?

ANDY: Well, they're sort of pornographic, these messages.

HELEN: So what you're telling me is that pictures of yourself, with an erection, together with these lewd messages have been spread all over the internet. Is that what you're trying to tell me?

ANDY: Well...yes.

HELEN: You propositioned these women.

ANDY: Well not exactly.

HELEN: What do you mean...not exactly? Did you proposition these women, or didn't you?

ANDY: Well, yes. I mean...it was just talk. I never meant to go through with it. And not only that.

HELEN: Go on.

ANDY: The story's on the front page of all the morning papers.

HELEN: I see. Pictures of yourself...

ANDY: In some papers, yes, along with the messages.

HELEN: *(With a sickening feeling)* Oh, Andy...!

ANDY: I know, I know. It's just that...

HELEN: It's just that...what? Tell me! What?!

ANDY: You mustn't get so excited.

HELEN: Go on.

POLITICS AS USUAL

ANDY: It's just that you're not always here.

HELEN: Are you trying to tell me that the fault is mine? Is that what you're trying to tell me? That I'm to blame for leaving you behind, doing my job, going off to Israel or Afghanistan? Is that what you're trying to tell me?

ANDY: Now calm done, Helen. I'm not blaming you. You mustn't excite yourself.

HELEN: Are you really that weak?

ANDY: Well, yes, I guess I am. I don't know. Maybe I need help. I don't want to lose you, Helen. You're not going to leave me, are you? Please. I don't want to lose you.

HELEN: You poor, sick boy, you stand to lose much more than a wife. How can you possibly run for governor now? And what about your seat in the Senate?

ANDY: I know, I know. I've got to get ready. I've called a news conference. It's gotten to the point where I just can't ignore it.

HELEN: What are going to say?

ANDY: I'll deny it. I'll say those pictures are a fake.

HELEN: I see.

ANDY: I've got to go. Neil's coming by.

HELEN: Neil?! Neil Grady?

POLITICS AS USUAL

ANDY: He's the one that's organized this press conference.

HELEN: Why on earth did you consult Neil Grady?

ANDY: I didn't consult him. He volunteered to help. As a matter of fact, he was the only one.

HELEN: And what did Neil have to say?

ANDY: He thinks it would be a good idea for me to step aside.

HELEN: And give up your seat?

ANDY: I suppose so. Helen?

HELEN: What?

ANDY: Can you forgive me? I wasn't really unfaithful. I never had anything to do with these women, not physically. Helen?

HELEN: What?!

ANDY: I never even met any of these women.

HELEN: And that makes it all right.

ANDY: No. No, of course not. I don't want to lose you. (*HE waits for a response.*) Helen?

HELEN: What?!

POLITICS AS USUAL

ANDY: Are you going to leave me?

HELEN: Andy, please. I need time to think about this.

ANDY: I'll do anything you say. Just don't leave me, Helen, please. I love you.

HELEN: Andy, please!

ANDY: Okay, okay.

(ANDY hesitates, then goes off. HELEN shakes her head in disbelief. SHE goes to the bar and, with trembling hands, pours a Scotch. SHE is about to down it.)

HELEN: What the hell am I doing? *(SHE sets the Scotch aside, at a loss for what to do next. After a moment, she goes to the phone and dials.)* Claire, is Howard there? Yes, it is, rather. Thank you. *(After a moment)* Howard? You've heard about it. I can't believe it! What sort of an idiot am I married to? *(SHE half laughs, half cries.)* Apparently. There's something so childish about the man. So "Needy" he calls it. What's that? The president? Oh, I'm so sorry. I'll let you go. No, no, no. I'll be all right. Thank you, dear.

(SHE hangs up, stands lost and confused, then sits, lost in thought ANDY reenters, wearing a tie and his suit jacket. HE stands studying her.)

ANDY: If you want to leave me, I'll understand.

HELEN: What are you going to say, at this news conference?

315

ANDY: I'll deny it. I'll say the pictures are a fake.

HELEN: And you think they'll believe you?

ANDY: You're disgusted with me.

HELEN: Andy, my sweet, don't you understand? It's not only you. This reflects on me. This reflects on Howard. This reflects on everyone connected with us.

ANDY: You mustn't upset yourself.

HELEN: What?

ANDY: When is it due?

HELEN: What? Five months from now.

ANDY: I don't want you getting all worked up. If you want to leave me, I'll understand.

HELEN: I heard you the first time! I understand that you'll understand! How many women were there, by the way?

ANDY: What's that? Four or five.

HELEN: Which is it, four or five?

ANDY: I don't remember?

HELEN: Have you been in touch with any of these women...I mean since it all came out? Have you any idea what they're going to say? I'm sure they've been contacted.

ANDY: I don't know.

HELEN: When I think that the president of the United States was at our wedding...and the Secretary of State...and the Vice President. And what about your family? Have you heard from any of them?

ANDY: Michael called.

HELEN: And what did your brother have to say?

ANDY: "I told you so."

HELEN: I suppose I should appear at your side, at this news conference I mean, but I'm just not up to it, Andy. I'm sorry. It was a long trip, and I'm absolutely exhausted.

ANDY: No, no, no. I don't expect you to.

HELEN: But denying that the pictures are false...is ridiculous.

ANDY: I've had calls this morning from some of my colleagues.

HELEN: And what did they have to say?

ANDY: A couple of them have been supportive.

HELEN: And the others?

ANDY: They want me to resign. What are you thinking?

POLITICS AS USUAL

HELEN: I'm just trying to understand. What sort of a man am I married to? What sort of a man is going to be the father of my child? Andy, you are a creep.

ANDY: Okay, okay.

HELEN: It is not okay. My God! You have had such a promising career. All that you've gone through; that uphill battle for that Senate seat. And all the plans we've been making. There was no doubt in my mind that you would have been elected governor. Haven't you got any self control? When you let yourself go like that, did you give no thought whatsoever to the consequences? Everything you've worked for, everything you've stood for. When are you due at this news conference?

ANDY: In an hour or so. (*HE looks at his watch.*) An hour and twenty minutes. What do you think I ought to do?

HELEN: Tell the truth. That's what I think you ought to do. Tell the truth and apologize.

ANDY: You don't think I should take a leave of absence?

HELEN: And give up your seat? No! Certainly not! You apologize, and you say that you will work twice as hard to make up for your mistakes. Look, I've said all I've had to say. I've had a long flight. I'd like to unpack and take a hot bath and relax. (*SHE rises, picks up her suitcase and starts off.*)

ANDY: Helen...

HELEN: What?

POLITICS AS USUAL

ANDY: I'll come right home afterwards. Helen...

HELEN: What? What is it?

ANDY: I said I'd come right home...

HELEN: I heard what you said.

ANDY: Will you be here?

HELEN: Will I be here? This happens to be my home. "Will I be here!"

ANDY: I don't want to lose you, Helen. Are you going to leave me?

HELEN: I see. Now that the cat's out of the bag, you're concerned about me. I don't want to hear another word!

(SHE goes off.)

ANDY: (HE sits with a sigh, and speaks half to himself.) As a matter of fact, I thought about you all the time.

(HELEN reenters. ANDY jumps up.)

ANDY: Yes? What is it?

HELEN: You said you're expecting Neil.

ANDY: He's going to pick me up.

HELEN: I'd like to speak to Neil before you leave.

ANDY: Okay.

(SHE goes off. ANDY sits, waiting nervously. After a moment, the doorbell rings. HE jumps up, then goes off to the foyer. NEIL GRADY, a beefy, businesslike man in his late forties enters with an attache case, followed by ANDY.)

NEIL: How are you doing?

ANDY: Helen's back.

NEIL: Oh? How did it go? The meeting...in Jerusalem?

ANDY: What? Oh. So, so. Nothing much was accomplished, I gather.

NEIL: If Howard had some balls... Ah well. You ready?

ANDY: As ready as I'll ever be.

NEIL: Just make it short and sweet. I've jotted down some notes.

(NEIL opens the attache case and takes out a sheet of paper, which he hands to ANDY, who looks it over.)

NEIL: Take your time. There's no rush.

(ANDY looks up, disturbed)

NEIL: What is it?

POLITICS AS USUAL

ANDY: Helen seems to think I shouldn't give up my seat.

NEIL: Oh?

ANDY: She thinks it would be a mistake.

NEIL: Well, I suppose she's thinking as a wife, as a woman who's in love with you.

ANDY: Yes, well I'm not so sure about that.

NEIL: About what?

ANDY: That she's in love with me. As a matter of fact...I think she's thinking about leaving me. And I really can't blame her. How could I have been so stupid?

NEIL: We're all of us human, old boy, and one doesn't always lead with one's head.

ANDY: You really think I should give up my seat?

NEIL: I think you've got to step back, give yourself some slack. In addition to that, you've got to think about the party. We certainly don't need this kind of distraction. As a matter of fact, there are several seats up for grabs and, as it is, old boy, we stand a good chance of losing the majority in the Senate, And, if you must know, I've spoken to the president.

ANDY: Oh? What did the president have to say?

NEIL: At first, it was "no comment", but then he added, "However, if I were Andy, I'd resign." (*HE looks at his watch.*) I think we'd better get going. You were going to say something.

ANDY: *(HE rises.)* No.

(THEY start off, then ANDY stops.)

NEIL: What is it?

ANDY: Helen wanted to talk to you before we left.

NEIL: Oh? Why don't you go on ahead. We're behind as it is. *(HE places his hand on ANDY'S shoulder.)* Go on. I'll be right behind you.

ANDY: Thank you, Neil. I really appreciate this.

NEIL: Go on, go on.

> *(NEIL pats him on the shoulder. ANDY goes off. NEIL heaves a sigh, then goes to the doorway leading to the interior.)*

NEIL: Helen?

HELEN: *(Offstage)* Just a minute.

> *(After a moment HELEN enters, wearing an attractive dressing gown.)*

NEIL: There she is, the sexiest aide a man ever had.

HELEN: Where's Andy?

NEIL: He went on ahead. He said you wanted to speak to me. How did things go?

HELEN: They went nowhere. And how are **your** plans shaping up? I understand you're gearing up to run for governor.

NEIL: Yes, well, it has crossed my mind.

HELEN: And has it crossed your mind that with Andy out of the way the path is clear?

NEIL: Helen, my dear, you and I both know that the path, in politics, is never clear. You baffle me, you really do. Why a woman as attractive as you are, as intelligent as you are...

HELEN: I'm listening.

NEIL: And as experienced in the ways of the world as you are...

HELEN: Go on.

NEIL: Would choose a man, or rather an overgrown boy, as foolish as your present husband.

HELEN: When I could have chosen....you?

NEIL: The trouble is, you're afraid of a real man, so you went out and chose yourself a weak little boy, well, maybe not so little, I gather. You're not going to stick it out, are you, this foolish marriage of yours? Look, you've made a mistake. Admit it. But the door's still open, Sweetie. Think about it.

We'd make a great team, you and I. You found me fascinating once.

HELEN: Neil, we dated a couple of times.

NEIL: More than a couple of times. Get rid of him.

HELEN: And then what?

NEIL: Marry me. What are you laughng at?

HELEN: I was just wondering what Mavis would have to say about that.

NEIL: I'll get rid of her. That was my mistake, and it was all your fault. That's right. You turned me down, and I married Mavis on the rebound.

HELEN: You are shameless.

NEIL: You've only yourself to blame. If only you weren't so godamned sexy, and there's that mind of yours that goes along with it. There ought to be a law against women like you.

HELEN: *(SHE laughs.)* Oh, Neil. I'm pregnant, you know.

NEIL: I'll adopt him.

HELEN: Are you really proposing?

NEIL: I never say anything I don't mean.

(SHE laughs.)

NEIL: All right, all right. I've got to go. Think about it. And, by the way, it might interest you to know what the president said.

HELEN: And what did the president say?

NEIL: "If I were him, I'd resign."

HELEN: I see.

NEIL: I've got to go. God, I'd give anything to have you on my side. Well, almost anything. *(HE takes her hand and kisses it.)* Think about it.

> *(HE goes off. SHE stands lost, deep in thought, sighs then starts off. The telephone rings. SHE hesitates then picks up the phone.)*

HELEN: Hello? Oh, Howard. No, he's gone. He's holding a news conference. I wanted him to stick it out. But I'm beginning to have second thoughts. *(After a moment.)* No, I'm not going to leave him. And besides, you've said yourself, that I'm going to make a splendid mother. Well, here's my chance, in spades; an overgrown boy to look after, and a child as well. *(SHE laughs.)* I know, I know

> *(The light has narrowed to a spot on HELEN, then fades.)*

KIDDING AROUND
A Play In One Act

CAST OF CHARACTERS
Harry Garrison
Fred Owens
Bonnie Webster
Mrs. Garrison

SCENE
Harry's room
A small town in the Midwest

(Late afternoon. HARRY, a handsome boy of seventeen, is seated at his computer, playing a game. FRED, an awkward boy of seventeen, appears in the open doorway, knocks on the door and enters the room.)

HARRY: You're back. What was it like?

FRED: Very emotional. Her mother broke down, and her aunt.

HARRY: What about her father?

FRED: He just looked somber, and sort of scary.

HARRY: Was there a big crowd?

FRED: Are you kidding? The whole town turned out. You should have been there. People asked about you.

HARRY: I just couldn't face it.

FRED: It made it look as if you didn't care. It wasn't your fault, Harry. We were all of just kidding around.

HARRY: If I hadn't nailed her, none of this would have happened.

FRED: (After a moment) What are you doing?

HARRY: This stupid game.

FRED: Which one is it?

HARRY: The motorcycle gang.

FRED: I don't have that one.

HARRY: Don't waste your money.

KIDDING AROUND

FRED: *(After a moment)* Have you decided which college you're going to apply to?

HARRY: No.

FRED: *(After a moment)* Are you okay?

HARRY: I had to take a sleeping pill.

FRED: You gotta be careful, Harry. They can be addictive. Bonnie's the one. She's the one that's responsible for all of this. She was the one who talked you into it.

HARRY: And like a damned fool, I let her. Showing off what a great cocksman I am. I should have listened to you..

FRED: Bonnie's always been a trouble maker. I really don't know what you see in her, Harry.

HARRY: She can be a lot of fun, when she wants to be.

FRED: Well, her sense of fun and mine are completely different. All right look, so you got the girl into bed. You didn't know what Bonnie had in the back of that stupid mind of hers. Putting that dildo into Jennie's locker. I'm sure she was the one.

HARRY: She says she wasn't.

FRED: That's what she says, and all those whistles and those hissing sounds. It was really too much. However, you must admit that Jennie Chomsky was not all there.

HARRY: She was a very intelligent girl.

FRED: Look, no sane person commits suicide. It's a scientific fact, and if it hadn't been us, something else would have come along.

KIDDING AROUND

From the moment I laid eyes on that girl, I knew there was something peculiar about her.

HARRY: She was shy.

FRED: Shy my foot! She acted like she was better than everybody else.

HARRY: Jennie was a nice, sweet kid, and very artistic. (*HE sighs, leaves the computer and sits in a chair with a sigh. After a moment...*) What about you? Have you decided...about college?

FRED: My father keeps talking about me helping him out in the store. And besides, my grades aren't really that good.

HARRY: You could probably get into State College.

FRED: I'm still thinking about it.

HARRY: I've had second thouhts.

FRED: Hey, now look, Harry, you're not gonna let this get you down?

HARRY: It's not only that. I'm thinking that maybe I'd be better off just settling down in town, and getting some kind of a job maybe.

FRED: What kind of a job?

HARRY: I don't know. Working in the post office maybe. I hear they're hiring all sorts of people.

FRED: After all that talk about politics, and the law, and everything? I'll betcha you could end up being a congressman, or even a senator maybe. I mean with the grades you got, and the fact that you're the captain of the swimming team, and your appearance.

KIDDING AROUND

Appearance means a lot, you know. I'll betcha you could get a scholarship to any college you chose. But you've gotta start now, Harry. At least a year ahead of time.

HARRY: *(After a moment)* Did you talk to Bonnie...at the funeral?

FRED: I don't talk to Bonnie, unless I absolutely have to. You should have seen her, carrying on as if she really cared. What a phoney she is?

HARRY: I'm sure she feels bad.

FRED: She doesn't feel anything, except maybe scared, since she was the ringleader.

HARRY: I got a call from Mr. Chomsky this morning.

FRED: Oh? What did he have to say?

HARRY: He said he wanted the truth.

FRED: What did you say?

HARRY: What could I say? I told him that sometimes some of us kidded around and, apparently, Jennie took things a little too serious maybe. He said that that was not the way he heard it. And then I told him about Mr. MacDonald, how he called us into his office, and how we had a long, long talk.

FRED: And what did he say?

HARRY: He called Mr. MacDonald an asshole, and he said that he was holding him responsible, as well as the faculty of the school, as well as some of the students.

FRED: Did he mention any names?

KIDDING AROUND

HARRY: No. But he said that there was gonna be a thorough investigation. And then he asked me if I had sex with his daughter.

FRED: Holy cow! What did you tell him?

HARRY: What could I say, since I was the only friend Jennie had at school?

FRED: Why did he think that you had sex with Jennie?

HARRY: 'Cause he found out that Jennie was not a virgin.

FRED: How did he find that out?

HARRY: From the autopsy.

FRED: Holy cow! Well, having sex isn't a crime, is it, especially if it isn't consensual, I mean if it is consensual.

HARRY: They can accuse me of raping her. They only have my word for it.

FRED: Who's gonna do the investigating? Did he say?

HARRY: The police, I guess.

FRED: (*After a moment*) Don't you have a swimming session this afternoon?

HARRY: It was called off.

FRED: I guess the whole town's been closed down. Everybody was at the funeral, and that's all that everyone is talking about; how these people came from a country where people were being oppressed, and that here in America we're supposed to be so open, so democratic. It was a crying shame, Mrs. Baxter said, and somebody's gotta be held responsible.

> *(THEY sit silently. After a moment, BONNIE, an attractive, bright looking seventeen year old appears in the doorway, knocks on the open door and enters.)*

BONNIE: *(To FRED)* Where did you disappear to?

FRED: They buried her, didn't they?

BONNIE: Everyone went to the house. They always serve food after a funeral. You should have come, Harry. You were the only student that wasn't there. Harry, the girl is dead.

HARRY: That's right, Bonnie. The girl is dead, and we are responsible.

BONNIE: *(After a moment)* Don't you have a swimming session this afternoon?

HARRY: It was called off.

FRED: Everything's been called off.

BONNIE: Who's asking you, sweetie pie?

HARRY: Okay, okay. Let's knock it off.

FRED: *(After a moment)* Harry says that Mr. Chomsky told him that there's going to be an investigation.

BONNIE: An investigation? Did you tell him about how Mr. MacDonald called us into his office, how he lectured us, and kept us there for hours?

KIDDING AROUND

HARRY: Of course, I did.

BONNIE: And what did he say?

HARRY: He called Mr. MacDonald an asshole. In addition to that, he's aware of the fact that I had sex with Jennie.

BONNIE: How did he find out?

HARRY: From the autopsy.

BONNIE: Is that what they do at an autopsy? Test your virginity?

FRED: Yeah. If you die tomorrow, your secret is out.

HARRY: Okay, Fred.

BONNIE: Well, even if there is an investigation, there wasn't any crime committed.

FRED: For your information, cruelty happens to be a crime.

BONNIE: What are you, nuts?

FRED: Harassment.

BONNIE: Well, we're under eighteen, so they can't charge us as an adult, that's if they can really charge us with anything. At any rate, just in case, this cousin of my father's a big time lawyer in Chicago..

FRED: Well, the way things look like now, you may be able to throw a lot of business his way.

BONNIE: What are you, some sort of a creep? Are you getting a kick out of all this?

KIDDING AROUND

HARRY: Will you two cut it out!

FRED: It's all her fault. Putting a dildo in her locker.

BONNIE: I did not put that dildo there.

FRED: Who did?

BONNIE: How the hell should I know?

FRED: And who was the one who gave her the idea to kill herself, drawing that sick picture of a girl with a rope around her neck.

BONNIE: Did she hang herself?

FRED: So she took some pills instead. But you were the one that planted the idea in her head.

HARRY: Okay, Fred. That's enough.

(THEY sit silently.)

BONNIE: Did you send in your application?

HARRY: What?

BONNIE: Your application to Princeton?

HARRY: No.

BONNIE: What are you waiting for? I sent in mine.

FRED: You're going to Princeton?

BONNIE: No, Sweetie. I'm going to Vassar.

KIDDING AROUND

HARRY: Did Mr. Chomsky say anything to you at the funeral?

BONNIE: He came up to me at the house.

HARRY: And what did he say?

BONNIE: He was really angry.

HARRY: What did you tell him?

BONNIE: I told him the same thing we told Mr. MacDonald. I told him that sometimes we used to tease Jennie, but it was all in fun. And he asked me if I knew that Mrs. Chomsky went in to see Mr. MacDonald a couple of weeks ago. Apparently Mrs. Chomsky was concerned about the way Jennie was behaving. And I said no, I didn't know anything about it.

HARRY: And then what did he say?

BONNIE: He didn't have a chance say anything. All sorts of people kept coming up to talk to him.

HARRY: You shouldn't have drawn that picture.

BONNIE: Oh, come on, Harry. The girl was not all there.

HARRY: Jennie was fine, until we started to go after her. Didn't I tell you that that drawing was not a good idea?

BONNIE: Yeah, after the fact. And when it comes to that, Harry, I did not force you to go to bed with her.

HARRY: And all that name-calling and cat whistles. She came to me in tears. She couldn't eat. She couldn't sleep. And she asked me if I couldn't put a stop to it.

KIDDING AROUND

BONNIE: As far as that's concerned, Jennie had her eyes on you the moment she saw you. *(SHE looks at FRED.)* What are you giggling at?

FRED: Of course, she had her eyes on him the moment she saw him. How else could she see him?

HARRY: Will you two, stop it!

FRED: She's the one that started it. She's always implying that I'm gay.

HARRY: So what if you are?

FRED: I'm not.

HARRY: So relax.

(THEY remain silent.)

BONNIE: *(After a moment)* Harry, there is no reason for you to get all worked up like this. Look, maybe we did go a little too far, but tell me honestly, did we deliberately set out to make Jennie kill herself? Did we? All right then. I'm not saying that we can't feel sorry for the girl. But the fact of the matter she is dead, and we've got our whole life ahead of us. I'll talk to my father, and he'll have a talk with Mr. Gottfried.

FRED: Who is Mr. Gottfried?

BONNIE: I told you. He's this big time lawyer in Chicago. *(To HARRY)* Did you send her any Emails?

HARRY: What?

BONNIE: Did you send her any Emails?

KIDDING AROUND

HARRY: We kept in touch by Email.

BONNIE: Do you remember what you wrote?

HARRY: I can look it up.

BONNIE: It might be a good idea to erase some of it. What have you got on there now?

HARRY: It's that new game.

BONNIE: Get rid of it

HARRY: Now?

BONNIE: No. Ten years from now.

HARRY: Well, hold on. *(HE sets aside the game and starts to bring up the record of his mail.)* What do you want to check?

BONNIE: The ones you sent her, to begin with.

HARRY: Hold on. *(HE brings up the mail he sent.)*

BONNIE: What did she call herself?

HARRY: Titania. She's queen of the fairies in Midsummer Nights Dream.

BONNIE: I know who Titania is. I'm not an idiot. And you're Oberon? Hold it. I'd like to read that one. *(SHE reads the letter.)* Were you in love with her?

HARRY: She was really very sweet.

BONNIE: You didn't tell me that you were in love with her.

KIDDING AROUND

HARRY: I wasn't in love with her.

FRED: That was the idea, wasn't it, Bonnie?

BONNIE: And she was in love with you, just like Fred

HARRY: I want you to stop it, here and now. You know, Bonnie, you really are a vicious person, and I'm sorry I ever got involved with you. And if you're not gonna stop picking on Fred, you can leave right now.

BONNIE: Okay, okay.

HARRY: What is it with you? I'd like to know. You make nasty cracks about everybody.

BONNIE: I'm sorry. All right?

HARRY: No, it isn't all right. I'd like to know what's bothering you?

BONNIE: There's nothing bothering me. And it just so happens that I happen to have feelings, just like everyone else.

HARRY: Well, you sure don't act like it. If you have a problem, Bonnie...

BONNIE: I haven't got a problem.

FRED: Would you like me to leave?

HARRY: No. Bonnie and I have had sex, which everyone knows. But we haven't made any sort of commitment. Have we?

BONNIE: Not really, no.

KIDDING AROUND

HARRY: Then tell me what's bothering you?

FRED: We've all of us got problems, Harry.

(BONNIE throws FRED a grateful glance.)

HARRY: Okay, okay. What do you want to do about the Emails?

BONNIE: What?

HARRY: The Emails. Bonnie?

BONNIE: It's been a long day, and that funeral took a lot out of me. I need a weed. *(She starts to open her purse.)*

HARRY: You can't smoke here.

BONNIE: Open a window.

HARRY: Bonnie!

BONNIE: Okay, okay.

(Mrs. Garrison, a well dressed, intelligent woman in her early forties, appears in the doorway and knocks on the open door. SHE holds a letter in her hand.)

MRS. GARRISON: Am I interrupting?

HARRY: No, no. Come on in. I understand the whole town turned out for the funeral.

MRS. GARRISON: Just about.

HARRY: I guess Mr. and Mrs. Chomsky were pretty upset.

KIDDING AROUND

MRS. GARRISON: Mrs. Chomsky had to be sedated. Jennie was her only child, you know.

HARRY: Did Mr. Chomsky say anything to you about an investigation?

MRS. GARRISON: As a matter of fact, we had a long talk about it.

HARRY: Who's we?

MRS. GARRISON: Mr. Chomsky, myself, as well as members of the school faculty. A couple of people insisted that there should be an investigation followed by a trial.

BONNIE: A trial?

MRS. GARRISON: Yes, a trial, a trial for those who took an active part in the hazing. Mr. Chomsky, in particular, was adamant about it. However, there is not going to be a trial. We were able to talk him out of it. There's going to be a town meeting instead.

HARRY: A town meeting?

MRS. GARRISON: Yes dear, a town meeting. The purpose of the meeting is to clear the air, to get things out in the open. You see, my dears, when one person dies, there are a lot of people who are affected. Jennie had relatives, here in America, as well as in the old country. There were people at the funeral who came all the way from Yugoslavia.

BONNIE: Mrs. Garrison...

MRS. GARRISON: Yes, Bonnie?

BONNIE: We never meant Jennie any harm.

KIDDING AROUND

MRS. GARRISON: I'm sure you didn't. You were just kidding around, or so I've been told.

BONNIE: If we had known...

MRS. GARRISON: On Sunday afternoon, after church, there will be a meeting at the Town Hall, and you will all get a chance to explain; to explain, among other things, the vicious letters that were sent to Jennie on her computer. Those who sent those letters will be asked to step forward, with the assurance that there will be no punishment. It was decided that punishment would only produce more antagonism.

FRED: Mrs. Garrison...

MRS. GARRISON: Yes, Fred?

FRED: I didn't really take part in any of that. As a matter of fact, I told Harry this was not a good idea. Didn't I, Harry?

MRS. GARRISON: You spoke to him privately.

FRED: Well, yes.

MRS. GARRISON: You were an onlooker.

FRED: I guess you might say that.

MRS. GARRISON: And you did nothing to stop it.

FRED: I felt very uneasy.

MRS. GARRISON: But you kept that to yourself, except to confide in Harry.

FRED: Well, yes.

KIDDING AROUND

MRS. GARRISON: Well, that's what you can tell Jennie's family, and everyone else at the town meeting. Harry...

HARRY: Yes? What is it.

MRS. GARRISON: This note was found on Jennie's computer, and we printed it out. It's addressed to you. I think you should read it...out loud, my dear, because you're going to be asked to read it out loud at the town meeting.

HARRY: Must I?

MRS. GARRISON: Yes, Harry. Would you like me to read it to you?

HARRY: Please.

MRS. GARRISON: *(SHE takes the letter out of the envelope and reads it.)*
Dear Oberon,
"The World is too much with us, and so I must bid you a fond farewell. When I came to this country, I thought, 'This is paradise. This charming town. I could make friends here, and life would be different.' But then I found that life here, was no different than it was in my old country. And then you came into my life and, for one brief moment, you made me believe that life could really be beautiful."
HARRY: Must you?

MRS. GARRISON: You're going to have to read this, Harry, in front of all those people.

HARRY: Okay, okay.

MRS. GARRISON: Shall I continue?

KIDDING AROUND

HARRY: Please.

MRS. GARRISON. "The hours we spent together... I never thought I could ever find such happiness. But then suddenly things changed, and I find that you, too, have succumbed to the forces of evil. And I've been forced to face the fact that there is no escape, no matter what country you live in."

(HARRY breaks down and starts to sob.)

MRS. GARRISON: *(After a moment)* Apparently she did make an attempt to write more, but the rest was just gibberish. They found her slumped over in front of her computer.

(There is a long silence.)

MRS. GARRISON: The meeting on Sunday is called for three o'clock. I understand that the governor might be there. *(To HARRY.)* I'll leave this note for you to look over. And I think the three of you had better give some thought to what you're going to say at that meeting.

(MRS. GARRISON leaves the letter on the desk and goes off. HARRY walks to the desk and picks it up, then lays it down. BONNIE walks over to HARRY and puts her arms around him. FRED comes over and puts his arms around both of them. The lights come down as they stand, their arms around one another.)

FANCY MEETING YOU
A Play In One Act

CAST OF CHARACTERS
Jessica Cartwright
Patricia Collins
Dennis Cartwright

SCENE
A hotel room

PATRICIA: I really think you're out of your mind. Did you hear what I said?

JESSICA: Yes, dear.

PATRICIA: And this awful, dreary hotel room! Why?

JESSICA: I was afraid I might run into someone.

PATRICIA: Sit down. I said, sit down.

JESSICA: If you're going to lecture me, you can leave right now.

PATRICIA: I'm not going to lecture you. I just want you to think this thing through. Please, sit down.

(JESSICA sits with a sigh. PATRICIA sits beside her.)

PATRICIA: Now, tell me, seriously, what brought this on?

JESSICA: I'm lonely.

PATRICIA: You're lonely. You have two lovely children. Three lovely grandchildren. A charming husband.

JESSICA: Dennis? Charming?

PATRICIA: Well, he can be, when he wants to be.

JESSICA: "When he wants to be." Everyone has a life of their own. Bobby and Laurie are all grown up and married. They have children of their own. What do they need me for? And Dennis has his office, and his poker club.

PATRICIA: What about your friends, your best friend, Helena?

JESSICA: Helena passed away last week.

PATRICIA: I'm so sorry. She was a lovely women.

JESSICA: She wasn't a lovely woman. She was a silly ass, but she was a lot of fun, and she made me laugh. Aren't you ever lonely?

PATRICIA: Yes, of course, I am.

JESSICA: What do you do about it?

PATRICIA: I make myself a cup of tea, or a drink.

JESSICA: And that's enough? A cup of tea, or a drink?

PATRICIA: And I have my career.

JESSICA: What about love?

PATRICIA: I love you...

JESSICA: I'm your sister.

PATRICIA: I love my nieces. I love my nephews.

JESSICA: You know perfectly well what I mean!

PATRICIA: You mean romantic love? Good Lord, Jessie I've had three affairs.

JESSICA: And what about now?

FANCY MEETING YOU

PATRICIA: I need a respite.

JESSICA: Well, I don't. My life is empty, and I intend to do something about it.

PATRICIA: Corresponding with some stranger on the internet.

JESSICA: He's not a stranger. He's the man of my dreams, sensitive and imaginative and...

PATRICIA: And you've gleaned all this from a couple of Emails?

JESSICA: It's been more than a couple of Emails. It's been going on for almost a month now.

PATRICIA: Have you any idea what this man looks like, how old he is, what he does for a living?

JESSICA: That's what we're here to find out.

PATRICIA: Are you thinking about having an affair with this man?

JESSICA: Let the cards fall where they may. I'm in the autumn of my years and I want them to be rich and fulfilling.

PATRICIA: I assume that Dennis knows nothing about all of this.

JESSICA: What do you think this is all about? Dennis and I have nothing to say to one another.

PATRICIA: Have you thought about what you're going to do when you meet this...this mysterious person whom you know nothing about? It may not even be a man for, God's sake. It may be a woman, for God's sake, a lesbian maybe, or an ax murderer. Have you thought about that?

FANCY MEETING YOU

(There is a knock at the door.)

PATRICIA: Well? Aren's you going to open the door.

JESSICA: You open it.

PATRICIA: *(SHE rises with a sigh.)* Incidentally, whom is this person looking for?

JESSICA: Penelope. The wife of Odysseus. And he's Odysseus, returning from a long, long voyage.

PATRICIA: He must be just as mad as you are.

(There is another knock at the door.)

JESSICA: Patty, please!

> *(PATRICIA puts her palms together, looks up to the heavens, takes a deep breath and opens the door. DENNIS CARTWRIGHT, a pleasant looking man in his early sixties appears.)*

DENNIS: Patty?

PATRICIA: *(SHE starts to laugh, then laughs hysterically, and continues to laugh uncontrollably.)* Please, do come in.

> *(DENNIS enters the room, and PATRICIA closes the door. DENNIS looks from JESSICA to PATRICIA.)*

DENNIS: *(To JESSICA)* Is this some sort of a joke? *(To PATRICIA)* Was this your idea?

PATRICIA: Don't look at me.

FANCY MEETING YOU

DENNIS: Then what, may I ask, are you doing here?

PATRICIA: I'm, what you might call, the chaperone.

DENNIS: I see. Well, now that you two have had your fun..(*HE starts for the door.*)

PATRICIA: I wouldn't, if I were you.

DENNIS: Haven't the two of you accomplished what you set out to do?

PATRICIA: And what might that be?

DENNIS: Make a fool of me apparently? (*To JESSICA*) Why aren't you laughing too?

JESSICA: I am not amused. Oh go! Why don't you go!?

PATRICIA: I think I'm the one that ought to leave.

JESSICA & DENNIS: No, don't.

PATRICIA: Well, that's a good start. You both agree on something.

DENNIS: I can see where Patty could dream up something like this, but I should think that you would have had more sense.

PATRICIA: Wrong as usual, Dennis. I'm the sensible one. That's why I've never married. It's so much easier to call it quits, when the affair is over.

DENNIS: For your information, Jessie and I happen to be married, and the marriage, I can assure you, is far from over.

FANCY MEETING YOU

PATRICIA: The contract, perhaps, the papal blessing, or whatever you want to call it? Maybe not. The relationship, however, that's another matter entirely.

DENNIS: What do you know about relationships, flitting from...one man to another...?

PATRICIA: Watch it, Dennis. I might just give you a piece of my mind.

DENNIS: Do you think you can spare it?

JESSICA: Patty, maybe you had better leave.

PATRICIA: With pleasure. *(SHE picks up her bag, kisses JESSICA and starts off.)* If you need me, call me...on my cell phone. Good luck, dear. *(SHE kisses her, then turns to DENNIS and giggles.)* Odysseus! *(SHE laughs as SHE goes off.)*

DENNIS: It's amazing. That woman can give the illusion of sweetness, of sensitivity, on the stage that is. In real life, however, she's as hard as nails.

JESSICA: My sister happens to be a very fine woman, loving and loyal.

DENNIS: So how come she's had three failures?

JESSICA: She doesn't consider them failures. She's still friends with all her lovers. That's more that you can say for us.

DENNIS: We're husband and wife. What has friendship got to do with it?

JESSICA: Nothing, my dear. Absolutely nothing.

351

FANCY MEETING YOU

DENNIS: *(After a moment)* Don't you have anything better to do? Making a fool of me like that. Are you really that bored?

JESSICA: And you? All those fantastic adventures, all that derring-do. I never knew you were that well read.

DENNIS: There are lots of things you don't know about me. And is this the way you get your kicks? Trying to make a fool of people?

JESSICA: Dennis, for your information, I never thought for one moment that you were Odysseus.

DENNIS: Are you trying to tell me you were carrying on, or you thought you were carrying on with a perfect stranger?!

JESSICA: And what about you?

DENNIS: I was just curious, that's all. You've been so aloof these days.

JESSICA: I can't believe you said that. I've been aloof?! You come down to breakfast every morning, you sit down at the breakfast table and you bury yourself in that newspaper of yours

DENNIS: Jessie, from time immemorial, I have always sat down at the breakfast table and checked the morning paper.

JESSICA: Checked it, yes. But you never used to bury yourself in it.

DENNIS: What's there to talk about, since you don't seem to be the least bit interested in what I've been up to?

JESSICA: How in the world would I know what you've been up to since you never share things with me anymore.

FANCY MEETING YOU

DENNIS: I never share things with you anymore because you're not interested.

JESSICA: How can I be interestd, when we have nothing in common? As a matter of fact, you're closer to the children, than you are to me.

DENNIS: You're jealous of the children?

JESSICA: Oh, don't be an idiot! The fact of the matter is I don't know who I am, or what I am. Why am I here? Of what use am I?

DENNIS: You're my wife.

JESSICA: Is that who I am? Someone you turn to every once in a while...to make love, if that's what you want to call it; a grunt and a groan, and then you're fast a sleep.

DENNIS: Well, I do have to get up in the morning. And hey, don't knock it. How many people our age are as active as we are...sexually, that is?

JESSICA: I am a person, Dennis. I'm a human being.

DENNIS: (After a moment) What's eating you, Jessie?

JESSICA: I've been wondering if we were ever really in love. When we married, we were much too young to know what love really is.

(Silence)

JESSICA: (Continued) Apparently we have nothing to say to one another, nothing to offer one another.

DENNIS: Don't be ridiculous..

FANCY MEETING YOU

JESSICA: What? Tell me! What? What have I got to look forward to? My career as a mother is over. My career as a wife...is what? Looking after a house?

DENNIS: Making a home.

JESSICA: A home? For whom? A stranger I have sex with every once in a while? A stranger, whom I discover, on the internet no less, happens to be a completely different person?

DENNIS: That wasn't me. I mean... I was just...playing a role.

JESSICA: Isn't that what we do every day, Dennis, play a role? We play husband and wife. We play mother and father and, if we live long enough, we play grandparents. But that's not who we really are, Dennis...to begin with that is?

DENNIS: What in the world are you talking about?

JESSICA: We begin life as a child, Dennis, a child with all sorts of dreams.

DENNIS: Dreams...exactly.

JESSICA: But that's who we really are, deep down inside. The child who's curious, who's searching, and we need someone to share those dreams. Didn't you have your dreams when you were growing up?

DENNIS: Yes, of course, I had my dreams. I wanted to be a ball player. I wanted to be a pitcher.

JESSICA: And I thought about being an actress, and Patty beat me to it.

FANCY MEETING YOU

DENNIS: I think you would have made a fine actress, a much better one than Patty. I remember you in that scene in that acting class we took at Ohio State.

JESSICA: Amanda, in Private Lives.

DENNIS: That's it. Amanda in Private Lives.

JESSICA: I was good, wasn't I?

DENNIS: In addition to that you're prettier than she is. You don't regret not being an actress, do you?

JESSICA: Whenever I think about Bobby and Laurie, no dear, no. *(After a moment)* Maybe we ought to get a divorce.

DENNIS: Is that what you want?

JESSICA: Apparently we have no interests in common, except for the childen, and they're no longer dependant on us.

DENNIS: *(After a moment)* My vacation's coming up in June. You enjoyed our trip to Spain last year.

JESSICA: Is that what I'm supposed to look forward to, a trip to Spain, or London once a year?

DENNIS: Hey, don't knock it. How many couples can afford a trip abroad every year. *(Pauses)* You want me to give up the poker club? Is that it?

JESSICA: God no! How could you possibly go on living without your poker club?

DENNIS: You want me to go to the opera with you?

JESSICA: And make yourself miserable?

DENNIS: What **do** you want?

JESSICA: I want a friend. That's what I want. Now that Helena's gone, there's no one I can have fun with anymore, no one I can relate to. I thought, for one moment, that I'd actually found someone.

DENNIS: *(After a moment)* There's never been anyone else but you, Jessie. You know that.

JESSICA: *(After a moment)* Isn't tonight your poker night?

DENNIS: I thought that coming home to Penelope, from a long, long voyage, would prove to be much more interesting.

JESSICA: Did you...really?

(*HE kisses her.*)

JESSICA: What about taking tennis lessons?

DENNIS: Tennis, at our age?

JESSICA: You were always talking about taking tennis lessons.

DENNIS: I'm game, if you are. *(After a moment)* What about that acting group, the Gallery Players? I read where they're doing Private Lives.

JESSICA: Are they really? Would you be interested?

DENNIS: I would be, if you are. *(After a moment)* Of course, we might be a little too old for Private Lives, but there are other plays. What are you thinking?

FANCY MEETING YOU

JESSICA: I'm thinking about my computer.

DENNIS: What about it?

JESSICA: It's really the most marvelous invention.

(SHE kisses him as the lights come down.)

CPSIA information can be obtained at www.ICGtesting.com
Printed in the USA
BVOW04s1722041213

338096BV00001B/22/P